Veröffentlichungen aus der
Geomedizinischen Forschungsstelle
(Leiter: Professor Dr. Dr. h.c. mult. G. Schettler)
der Heidelberger Akademie der Wissenschaften

Supplement zu den Sitzungsberichten der
Mathematisch-naturwissenschaftlichen Klasse
Jahrgang 1991

W. Morgenstern M. S. Tschechkovski
E. Nüssel G. Schettler (Eds.)

CINDI
Countrywide Integrated Noncommunicable
Diseases Intervention Programme

Baseline Evaluation

With 23 Figures

A joint publication with

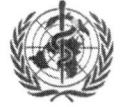 World Health Organization
Regional Office for Europe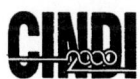

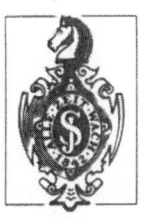 Springer-Verlag Berlin Heidelberg GmbH

Dipl.-Math. Wolfgang Morgenstern
Geomedizinische Forschungsstelle
Heidelberger Akademie der Wissenschaften
Karlstr. 4, W-6900 Heidelberg, FRG

Dr. Mark S. Tsechkovski
Regional Office for Europe, World Health Organization
Scherfigsvej 8, DK-2100 Copenhagen, Denmark

Prof. Dr. Egbert Nüssel
Abt. Klinische Sozialmedizin, Universitätsklinikum Heidelberg
Bergheimer Str. 58, W-6900 Heidelberg, FRG

Prof. Dr. Dr. h.c. mult. Gotthard Schettler
Geomedizinische Forschungsstelle
Heidelberger Akademie der Wissenschaften
Karlstr. 4, W-6900 Heidelberg, FRG

The views expressed in this book do not necessarily
represent the decisions of the stated policy of the
World Health Organization

ISBN 978-3-540-54646-7   ISBN 978-3-662-02686-1 (eBook)
DOI 10.1007/978-3-662-02686-1

© Springer-Verlag Berlin Heidelberg 1991
Originally published by Springer-Verlag Berlin Heidelberg New York in 1991.

Typesetting: Camera ready by author

Authors

D.R. MacLean,[1] A. Petrasovits,[2] I. Glasunov[3]
and H. Korhonen[4]

On behalf of the CINDI Collaborative Group:

Austria   H.- P. Bischof and R. Schiemer

Bulgaria   L. Ivanov

Canada   S. Stachenko

Czech and Slovak Federal Republic

                              J. Boukal

Finland   P. Puska and A. Nissinen

Federal Republic of Germany

                              E. Nüssel, W. Barth, W. Scheuermann
                              and W. Morgenstern

Hungary   R. Horvath, T. Kovacs and A. Szilasi

Iceland   P. Sigurdsson, O. Olafsson,
                              A. Grimsson, N. Sigfusson,
                              B. Thjodleifsson and H.V. Fridriksson

Israel   J.R. Viskoper, U. Gabbai, S. Rishpon
                              and A. Arditi

Malta	G. Galea
Portugal	F. de Padua, A. Coelho and B. da Costa
United Kingdom	A.E. Evans, J. Wilde and E. McCrum
USSR	R.G. Oganov
Byelorussia	G. Sidorenko, I. Kozlov and E. Zborovsky
Estonia	A. Ellamaa, N. Elshtein and O. Volozh

Industrial enterprises

V. Molchanov, A. Ivanov, R. Potyemkina and V. Lisitsyn

Lithuania	V. Grabauskas, I. Miseviciene and A. Baubiniene
Moscow	L. Chazova and G.S. Zhukovsky
Novosibirsk	Y. Nikitin and G. Simonova
Yugoslavia	M. Planojevic

WHO Regional Office for Europe

M. Tsechkovski, A. Shatchkute and A. Müller

1 Department of Community Health and Epidemiology, Faculty of Medicine, Dalhousie University, Nova Scotia, Canada
3 Health Promotion Directorate, Health and Welfare, Ottawa, Canada
3 WHO Regional Office for Europe, Copenhagen, Denmark
4 Department of Epidemiology, National Public Health Institute, Helsinki, Finland

Foreword

The WHO strategy for health for all, unanimously adopted by all Member States a decade ago, offers both a challenge and a powerful tool to turn the vision of people's health as an integral and inseparable part of overall social development into reality. Improving people's health involves not only the health services, with their predominantly curative function, but also all sectors responsible for creating health promotive social, economic, physical and cultural environments which can thus make healthy lifestyles the easy lifestyle to choose. This intersectoral principle has served as the basis for the innovative development of an integrated, multidisciplinary, community-based approach aimed at effectively controlling and reducing the prevalence of noncommunicable diseases. During recent decades, these have continued to pose a major health problem and be a cause for concern in industrialized countries.

This approach emphasizes promoting health and preventing disease through existing health care systems and the active participation of both communities and individuals. Its scope is thus broader than the traditional delivery of health by services alone; it promotes responsibility for health both in the individual and in the community, and its strategies are designed to facilitate change at both levels and in all sectors of society.

The countrywide integrated noncommunicable diseases intervention (CINDI) programme embodies these principles, representing a practical implementation of the health for all strategy in noncommunicable diseases in the European Region and in Canada.

The programme has gathered experience in developing the integrated prevention of noncommunicable diseases through primary health at the local level. This experience is beginning to have an impact at the country level in all the CINDI member countries.

This report addresses the issue of monitoring and evaluating programmes of this kind and presents some baseline data to illustrate this process.

G. Schettler   J.E. Asvall

Head   WHO Regional Director
Unit for Geomedical Research   for Europe
Heidelberg Academy for the
Humanities and Sciences

Contents

1 Introduction

The countrywide integrated noncommunicable diseases intervention (CINDI) programme is a major vehicle of the World Health Organization (WHO) in the European Region and is considered essential for the WHO regional policy for achieving health for all by the year 2000. CINDI focuses on the commonality of risk factors for noncommunicable diseases and intervention against these diseases, and sets targets and then conducts full scientific evaluation of how well these targets are being met. In addition, targeting intervention and evaluating intervention methods are a key part of CINDI. Intersectoral collaboration at all levels, from the lay public to governments, is crucial in ensuring its success. The initiation of the CINDI programme was largely based on the experiences gained in another European project coordinated by WHO: the comprehensive cardiovascular community control programme.[1]

The purpose of this report is to present selected data that will serve as the baseline for the long-term evaluation of the outcome of CINDI programmes both countrywide and in demonstration areas. The epidemiological indicators have been selected to reflect a common core that will serve as a basis for a comparative evaluation of CINDI programmes.

This report is not intended to serve as a comprehensive epidemiological overview of noncommunicable diseases in participating countries. The data presented here were collected according to the longitudinal CINDI evaluation design.

The baseline data follow up the *CINDI protocol and guidelines for monitoring and evaluation procedures* [2] (called *Guidelines* in this report). The *Guidelines* recommend a range of indicators and procedures for managing and evaluating programme interventions. They ensure standardization and comparability of data collection. This common approach should support the planning,

---

[1] Puska P (ed.) (1988) Comprehensive cardiovascular community control programmes in Europe. EURO Reports and Studies No. 106. WHO, Copenhagen
[2] Leparski E, Nüssel E (eds.) (1987) CINDI protocol and guidelines for monitoring and evaluation procedures. Springer, Berlin Heidelberg New York

implementation and evaluation of programme intervention and should enable the value of the approaches and intervention procedures used in CINDI countries to be assessed.

CINDI programmes have begun to implement the *Guidelines* in accordance with the specific circumstances in each country and the constraints on data availability. The programme directors in the participating countries have agreed on a basic core set of diseases and risk factor indicators to assess the long-term outcome of the programme.

In preparing this report the CINDI programme directors in each country, the CINDI Programme Management Committee, the CINDI Coordinating Centre and the CINDI Data Management Centre were consulted. WHO headquarters provided the mortality data. The risk factor data are from the baseline surveys carried out between 1982 and 1987 by the participating countries in the demonstration areas.

The indicators presented here as the core of the outcome evaluation have been identified in the *Guidelines*. Most CINDI centres collect data on a wider range of indicators than those presented here; they include, for example, data on accident incidence, the prevalence of diabetes and health inequalities.

The core indicators in this evaluation are the mortality rates and risk factors for the major noncommunicable diseases in industrialized countries. The baseline indicators selected are practical, as they represent data currently available in the participating CINDI countries that are sufficiently reliable to allow the assessment of the long-term impact of the programmes.

The European Region of WHO has set 38 targets for health for all. These targets provide a policy context, to CINDI and non-CINDI countries alike, for the development of countrywide intervention against noncommunicable diseases. The review of baseline indicators is directed towards the managers of CINDI programmes and the authorities in relevant jurisdictions in the participating countries.

This report is intended to assist in setting priorities for health policy and programme development and to facilitate the implementation of the three major complementary strategies that are available: health promotion, disease prevention and providing appropriate health services.

2 Preventing Noncommunicable Diseases: an Opportunity to Contribute towards Achieving Health for All

Noncommunicable diseases is a large category that encompasses a wide range of disorders. These include: diseases of the circulatory system, chronic respiratory diseases, cancer and trauma resulting from accidents. They are the major causes of mortality in developed countries. Ischaemic heart disease, cancer, cerebrovascular diseases (stroke), respiratory diseases, injury and poisoning account for about 80% of total deaths (Fig. 1).

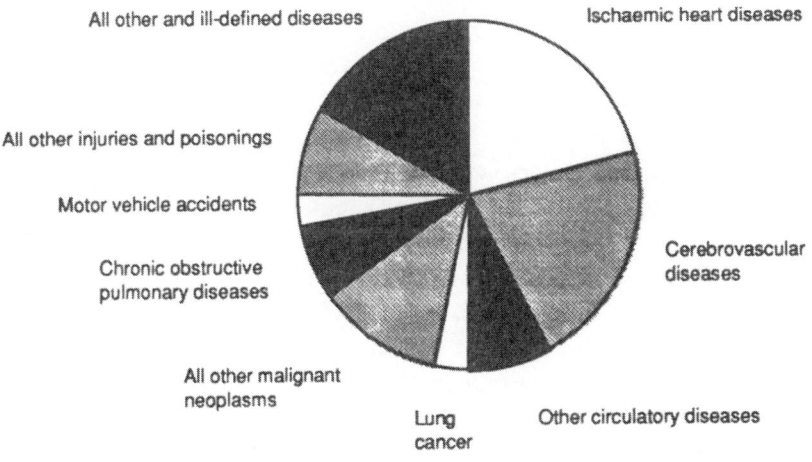

Fig. 1. Leading causes of death in developed countries (about 1986-1987). Source: World Health Organization (1989) World health statistics annual. Who, Geneva

The mortality rates for cardiovascular disease and some types of cancer have been declining in some countries in the last two decades. Nonetheless, noncommunicable diseases remain by far the main cause of premature mortality, morbidity and disability and account for the major part of health care expenditure.

The overall social cost of noncommunicable diseases is massive, and can be illustrated by their impact on years of life lost (Fig. 2). Accidents and poisoning, diseases of the circulatory system and cancer account for the bulk of years of life lost for people aged below 65 years.

Major gains in health can be achieved by effectively controlling noncommunicable diseases. The hallmark of most noncommunicable diseases is their multifactorial etiology. This is in contrast with some communicable diseases, which mainly require the presence of one infective agent and a susceptible host for their manifestation.

Most cardiovascular diseases and the common types of cancer can either be prevented or controlled by taking action on risk factors or by developing programmes for early identification of subclinical or clinical disease. Only a few factors account for the premature development of most of these diseases. For example, smoking and a diet rich in fat or high caloric intake along with low energy expenditure are responsible for much of the current epidemic of premature cardiovascular disease and lung cancer and for the high prevalence of such premorbid conditions as obesity, elevated blood pressure and elevated serum cholesterol.

The widespread prevalence of risk factors in industrialized countries resulting from unhealthy lifestyles is especially significant for prevention. Negative dietary habits, sedentary lifestyles, the use of tobacco, alcohol and drugs, and such social factors as alienation and lack of social support are related to living conditions. Most of the noncommunicable diseases and the attendant risk factors manifest themselves more often in the lower socioeconomic groups of the population.

The onset of the risk factors for most noncommunicable diseases occurs early in life, usually in childhood, when unhealthy lifestyle habits are first established, which emphasizes the need for prevention. The initial clinical manifestation of cardiovascular disease and of cancer often appears when the disease is far advanced. In many instances, the first symptoms of ischaemic heart disease coincide with sudden death. In these circumstances, a preventive approach is the most viable option for meaningful intervention. Treatment of these conditions is costly and the prognosis is often poor.

The risk factors common to most noncommunicable diseases are widespread. For example, in CINDI countries, approximately two-thirds of the population has one or more major risk factors for cardiovascular disease. Many people have a significantly increased risk of disease because of excessive levels of one risk factor or because several risk factors are moderately elevated, which may confer a high risk of disease. For example, the bulk of cardiovascular disease does not come from the clustering of high levels of risk in a small part of the

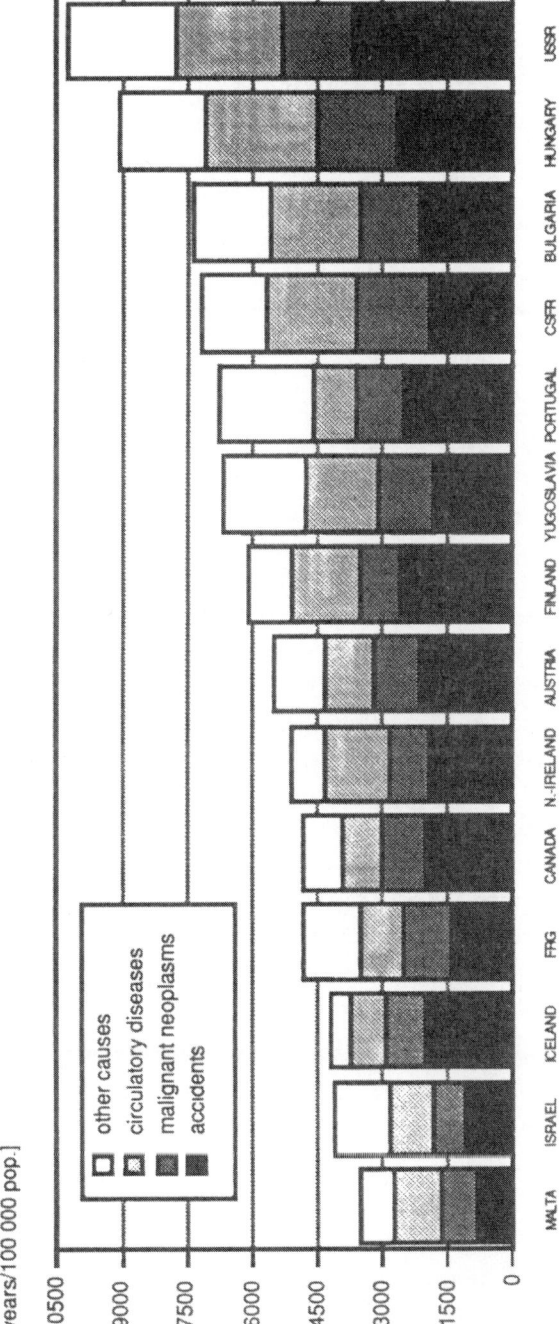

[years/100 000 pop.]

Fig. 2. Years of potential life lost (years per 100 000 population) for people 1-64 years old from injury and poisoning, diseases of the circulatory system, malignant neoplasms and from other causes (about 1987-1988). Source: World Health Organization (1989) World health statistics annual. Who, Geneva.

CSFR, Czech and Slovak Federal Republic; FRG, Federal Republic of Germany before 3 October 1990

population, but rather from a widespread prevalence of moderate levels of risk in the bulk of the population.

Appropriate primary and secondary health care services are required to identify high-risk individuals and to provide them with appropriate follow-up services, counselling and management. Inherent in the CINDI approach is the need for adequate coordination between the services and programmes directed towards high-risk groups and health promotion and education among the general population.

A number of neoplastic conditions can be detected at early stages of development. For some of these conditions, such as cervical and breast cancer, early identification is valuable for certain population groups. Appropriate and accessible services as well as health education programmes are needed to extend the benefits emerging from opportunities for early detection, control and treatment of noncommunicable diseases to the relevant target groups.

A balanced approach is required, including intervention directed towards the population as a whole and towards high-risk groups and people with clinical disease. Prevention and control thus require the commitment of the health care sector and of health professionals as well as multidisciplinary and intersectoral measures that create conditions conducive to healthy living by emphasizing the need for environmental changes. People live in communities and they therefore need to be encouraged to define issues that can be transferred to the community level. Encouraging community participation is a key strategy in setting priorities and in developing programmes to deal with them.

Inter-country comparisons of mortality rates and risk factors in CINDI countries (Chapter 4) suggest that important strides can be made in reducing mortality from noncommunicable diseases and in reducing the prevalence of attendant risk factors. Community intervention programmes and risk factor reduction trials have demonstrated the efficacy of health promotion and of preventing noncommunicable diseases. The declines in risk factor prevalence and mortality rates observed in a number of CINDI countries (Chapter 4) and other developed countries attest to the potential effect a broadly based health promotion approach can have on the health status of populations.

3 Evaluation Framework and Epidemiological Indicators for the First Baseline Evaluation

The *Guidelines* emphasize that the information system of every participating country should include an evaluation component. Evaluation should cover process and outcome measures. Process evaluation assesses the feasibility and performance of the programme: to what extent and how the planned activities are being implemented. Outcome evaluation focuses on how well the programme has reached its objectives, formulated in measurable terms using relevant indicators.

The breadth of the CINDI programme goals and the variety and complexity of its intervention procedures, which take place at different levels, pose a significant challenge in establishing an adequate comprehensive evaluation framework. Both the *Guidelines* and this report are a first step in the continuing development and implementation of this framework.

According to the CINDI programme, evaluation is needed in demonstration areas and countries and between countries. At each of these levels, the objectives of the programme are oriented towards the common goals of preventing and controlling noncommunicable diseases. Nevertheless, the programme objectives, strategies and activities as well as its purpose, the measures used and the expectations for evaluation vary for each of these levels. For example, legislation can be used at the country level to control the use of tobacco. Within demonstration areas, public education and persuasion are appropriate activities to further anti-smoking objectives. Evaluating the impact of these activities at the country level may involve countrywide surveys to monitor trends in smoking. Within demonstration areas, evaluation may involve monitoring smoking trends and initiatives to create nonsmoking areas at work and in public places.

The framework for evaluating CINDI programmes developed in the *Guidelines* includes measures for defining a comprehensive system, including evaluation needs at the demonstration area, country and inter-country levels.

The multifactorial etiology and the long incubation period of noncommunicable diseases makes it difficult, if not possible, to attribute change in disease outcome in the population to activities promoting prevention implemented in demonstration areas or even countrywide. Clinical intervention is targeted at the individual. The outcome may usually be determined in a period of months to a few years. Outcome evaluation typically assesses efficacy: whether the intervention works under ideal conditions. Using appropriate experimental designs, the attributability of the outcome to the clinical manœuvre may be established in terms of accepted scientific criteria of validity. It is usually practical to carry out this type of evaluation with limited financial resources and over a relatively short time.

By contrast, intervention directed towards communities in a demonstration area or towards a whole country does not provide the opportunity to study the relationship between intervention and outcome using traditional scientific criteria of validity. Documented examples in the literature show how major community intervention programmes involving public education campaigns targeted at a whole region are subject to the influence of programmes carried out elsewhere. The use of control areas in countrywide programmes is not feasible or desirable scientifically, financially or ethically.

The current evaluation framework for the WHO CINDI programme consists of the following elements, which are classified as essential outcome indicators in the *Guidelines* :

1. The age-standardized mortality rates and time trends for the major non-communicable diseases by gender for people aged 25-64 years:

    *   all-cause mortality;

    *   diseases of the circulatory system, including ischaemic heart disease and cerebrovascular disease;

    *   malignant neoplasms, including malignant neoplasms of the trachea, bronchus and lung (strongly related to smoking) and malignant neoplasms of the small intestine, duodenum and colon (strongly related to diet);

    *   diseases of the respiratory system; and

    *   chronic liver diseases and cirrhosis.

2. The age-standardized prevalence of major risk factors for major noncommunicable diseases by gender for people aged 25-64 years:

    *   elevated serum cholesterol

- elevated blood pressure

- elevated body mass index

- regular cigarette smoking

- the presence of one or more risk factors.

The risk factor data are available from special surveys carried out in the demonstration areas, and thus may not be representative of each country as a whole.

The age group 25-64 years was chosen for mortality rates and risk factor prevalence to establish a common core of data available in all participating CINDI countries. This age group is best suited for monitoring the effects of health promotion and disease prevention efforts.

In addition to these baseline indicators, for the common core evaluation of outcome, most countries participating in CINDI use other indicators of other major noncommunicable diseases that cover younger and older groups. Risk factor data other than those referred to above are being included in demonstration area surveys. Process evaluation measures have also been developed for use in CINDI programmes and will be the subject of a follow-up baseline report.

4 Overview of the Epidemiological Baseline Indicators

This chapter provides an overview of the baseline data on noncommunicable diseases and risk factor levels in the CINDI countries. Two types of data are given: mortality statistics and survey data on risk factors for major noncommunicable diseases (elevated blood pressure, elevated serum cholesterol, smoking and elevated body mass index). They represent the essential core evaluation indicators that have been collected for all the participating CINDI countries and centres.

The mortality statistics include total and disease-specific rates expressed as deaths per 100 000 people per year for men and women 25-64 years of age, standardized to the European standard population. The calendar year for which calculations are made is 1982 (for exceptions see Annex 7.3). The trends of the rates are expressed as the percentage change between 1973 and 1982.

The mortality rate data are presented for each country (CINDI member) to show the country's relative position. The analysis was made for the following CINDI member countries: Austria, Bulgaria, Czech and Slovak Federal Republic (CSFR), Federal Republic of Germany (FRG), Finland, Hungary, Iceland, Israel, Malta, Northern Ireland, Portugal and Yugoslavia. The data presented for the Federal Republic of Germany and the German Democratic Republic (GDR) apply to the countries before 3 October 1990. The German Democratic Republic was a full CINDI member before unification. The data on mortality from the USSR for 1973-1982 were not available, but data for Lithuania were provided.

Tables that present the data used in the figures in this chapter are presented in Annex 7.4.

The total mortality rates among men vary widely in the CINDI countries (Fig. 3). The lowest rate (Iceland) is less than half of the highest rate (Lithuania). The total mortality among men decreased by varying amounts in most of the countries, but Hungary, Lithuania, Bulgaria, Czechoslovakia and Yugoslavia had increasing rates. The mortality rates for diseases of the circulatory system were nearly proportional to total mortality rates, with some variation, and the mortality rates for cancer were very similar in all the countries.

Fig. 4 presents all-cause mortality for women from the same countries as well as ten-year trends. The rates among women 25-64 years of age were much lower than those of men. The rank order of the countries was different for women; for example, mortality was very low among women and high among men in Finland. Another important feature is that diseases of the circulatory system was not the major contributor to the overall mortality rate, as it was for men. Only Bulgaria, Hungary and Lithuania had no decrease in total mortality from 1973 to 1982; Lithuania and Hungary substantially increased and Bulgaria did not change.

Ischaemic heart disease (IHD) rates vary more widely between CINDI countries than do total mortality rates (Fig. 5). The highest IHD rates (Northern Ireland and Finland, 283 and 277 per 100 000, respectively) are more than three times higher than the lowest rates (Portugal and Yugoslavia, 75 and 96 per 100 000, respectively).

The ten-year trend shows an increase in Lithuania, Hungary, Bulgaria, Yugoslavia, Czechoslovakia, Malta and Austria. The rates declined in Canada, Finland, Israel, Iceland, FRG, Portugal, Northern Ireland and GDR (listed in order of decreasing decline). Although Finland had the greatest absolute decrease in mortality from IHD in men, the absolute rate of IHD stayed very high. To a lesser extent, the same was true of Canada.

The rank order of mortality rates from IHD in women (Fig. 6) is rather similar to that of men. The difference in mortality rates between countries is fourfold, ranging from 21 for Portugal to 81 for Northern Ireland. The absolute mortality rates are much lower among women than among men: 21-81 for women versus 75-283 for men. Only Lithuania, Hungary and Yugoslavia had an increase in the rates among women from 1973 to 1982. GDR and Czechoslovakia had no change and the other countries showed a decrease.

The mortality rates from cerebrovascular disease among men and women reveal a similar variation and rank order for the countries (Fig. 7 and 8). The rates for men range from 15 to 104 and, for women, 10 to 69, so that the absolute values are also similar for men and women. The rates in Hungary increased to a very high level from 1973 to 1982. The rates for both genders increased in Hungary, Lithuania and Bulgaria, and the rates for men increased slightly in Iceland and Yugoslavia. To varying degrees, the rates decreased in all of the other countries, especially among women.

The age-standardized mortality rates from malignant neoplasms of the trachea, bronchus and lung - cancers related to smoking - increased among both men and women in most of the CINDI countries (Fig. 9 and 10). Only Finland and Northern Ireland (men) and Bulgaria (women) experienced a substantial decrease in these rates. As in previous cases, the rates vary substantially between the countries.

Eight CINDI countries showed an increase in rates of malignant neoplasms of the small intestine, duodenum and colon among men and nine countries showed the same trend among women (Fig. 11 and 12). The trends in mortality rates were the same for men and women in most of the countries. These cancers are regarded as being related to diet.

The trends in mortality rates from respiratory diseases were very similar for men and women from 1973 to 1982 (Fig. 13 and 14). The rates for men and women very clearly decreased in all the CINDI countries, except in Hungary and Israel, where the rates increased for both men and women, and the rates for women increased in the GDR.

The mortality rates from chronic liver diseases and cirrhosis (Fig. 15 and 16) increased in most of the countries for both men and women from 1973 to 1982. The increase was especially high among both genders in Hungary, Bulgaria and Yugoslavia, and for men only in Northern Ireland.

The pattern of mortality indicators in CINDI countries shows that:

• The total and cause-specific mortality rates vary substantially between the countries, with a two- to fourfold difference between the extremes.

• For cardiovascular disease mortality, and specifically for ischaemic heart disease and cerebrovascular disease, the rates for 1973-1982 increased for most countries in eastern Europe and decreased variably for most of the other countries. Nevertheless, the absolute values remain high in all countries.

• The mortality rates from respiratory cancer increased from 1973 to 1982 among both men and women in most countries.

• The mortality rates from respiratory diseases decreased from 1973 to 1982 among both men and women in almost all countries.

• The mortality rates from chronic liver disease and cirrhosis increased from 1973 to 1982 among both men and women in most countries.

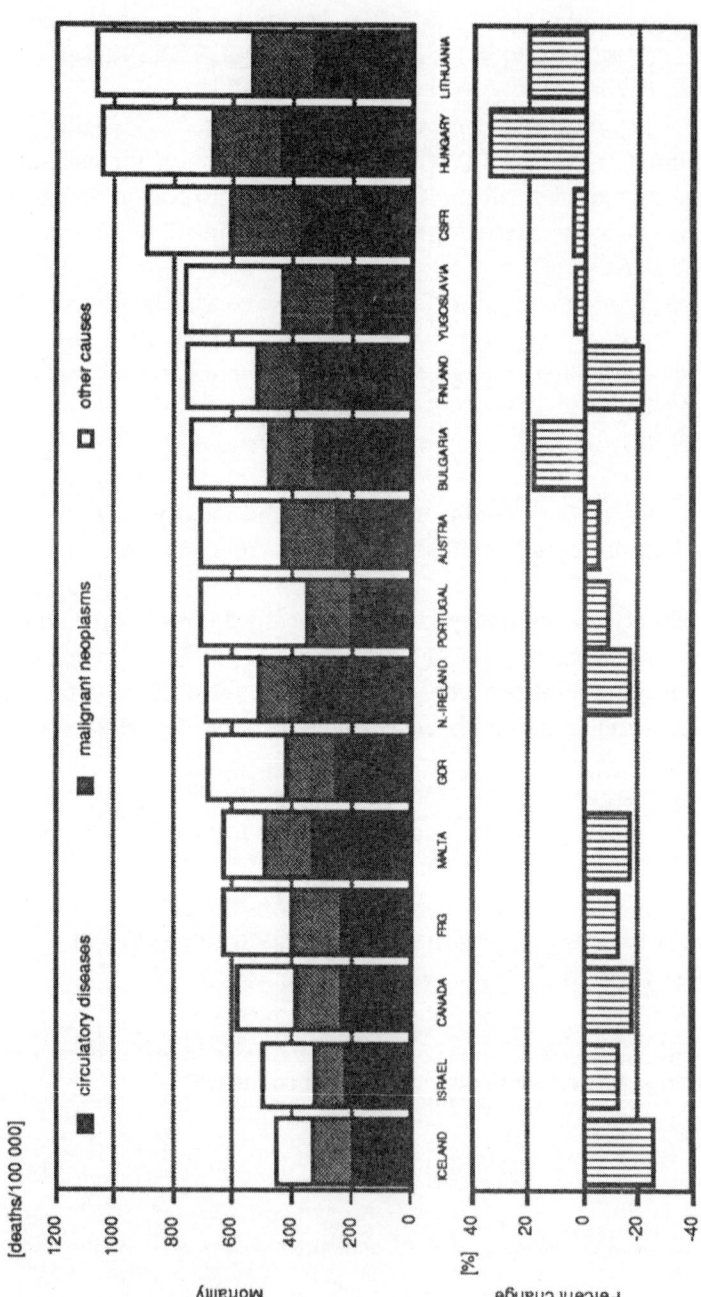

Fig. 3. Age-standardized all-cause mortality in 1982 from diseases of the circulatory system, malignant neoplasms as well as other causes and percentage change in all-cause mortality from 1973 to 1982 among men aged 25-64 years.

CSFR, Czech and Slovak Federal Republic; FRG, Federal Republic of Germany before 3 October 1990; GDR, former German Democratic Republic

15

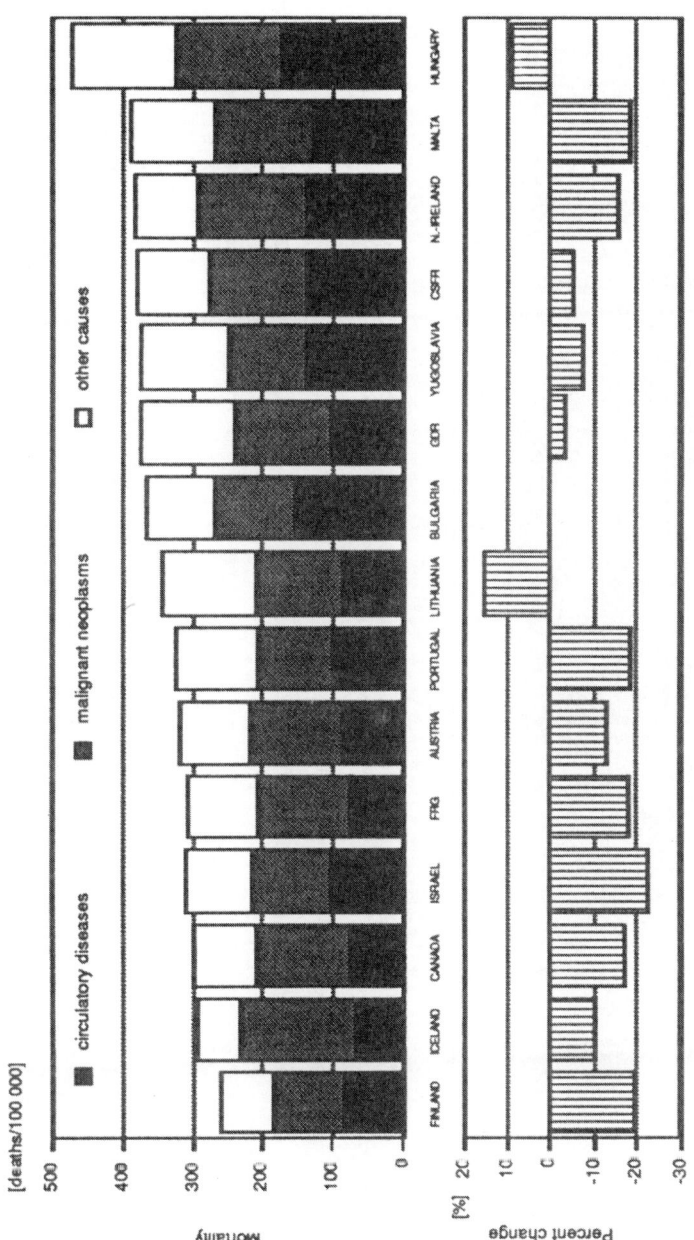

Fig. 4. Age-standardized all-cause mortality in 1982 from diseases of the circulatory system, malignant neoplasms as well as other causes and percentage change in all-cause mortality from 1973 to 1982 among women aged 25-64 years.

CSFR, Czech and Slovak Federal Republic; FRG, Federal Republic of Germany before 3 October 1990; GDR, former German Democratic Republic

16

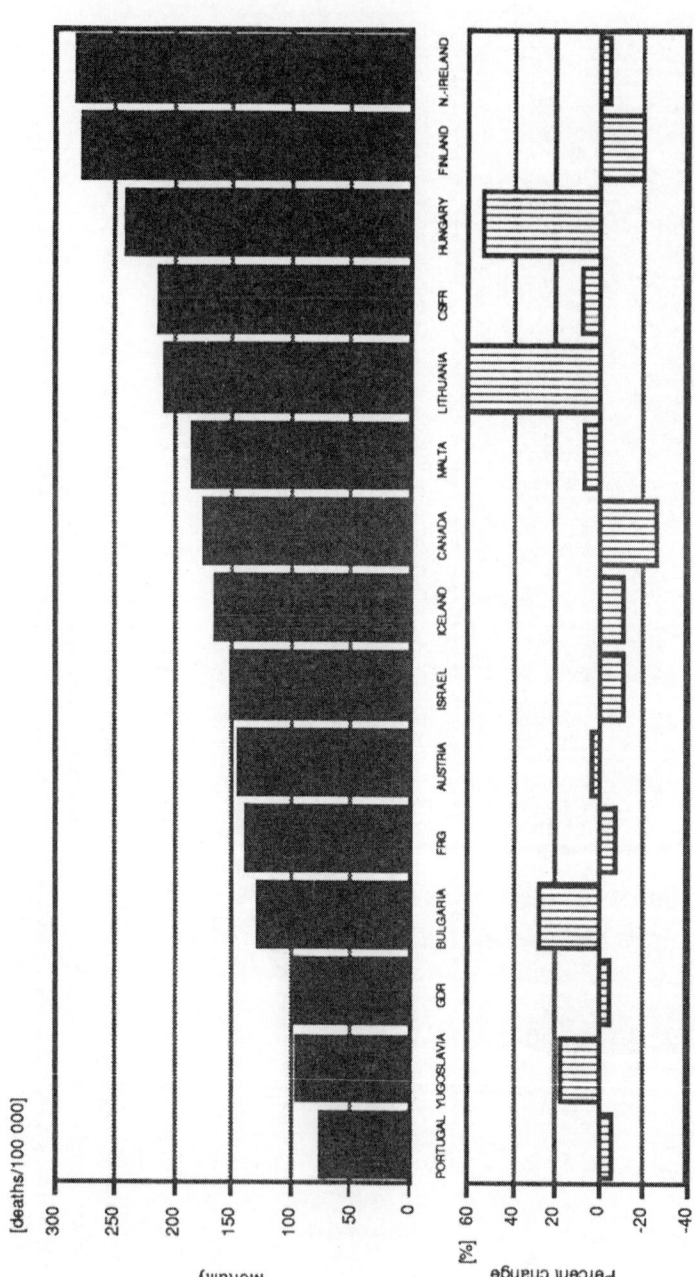

Fig. 5. Age-standardized mortality rates (deaths per 100 000 population) from ischaemic heart disease (ICD 410-414) and percentage change from 1973 to 1982 among men aged 25-64 years.

CSFR, Czech and Slovak Federal Republic; FRG, Federal Republic of Germany; GDR, former German Democratic Republic

17

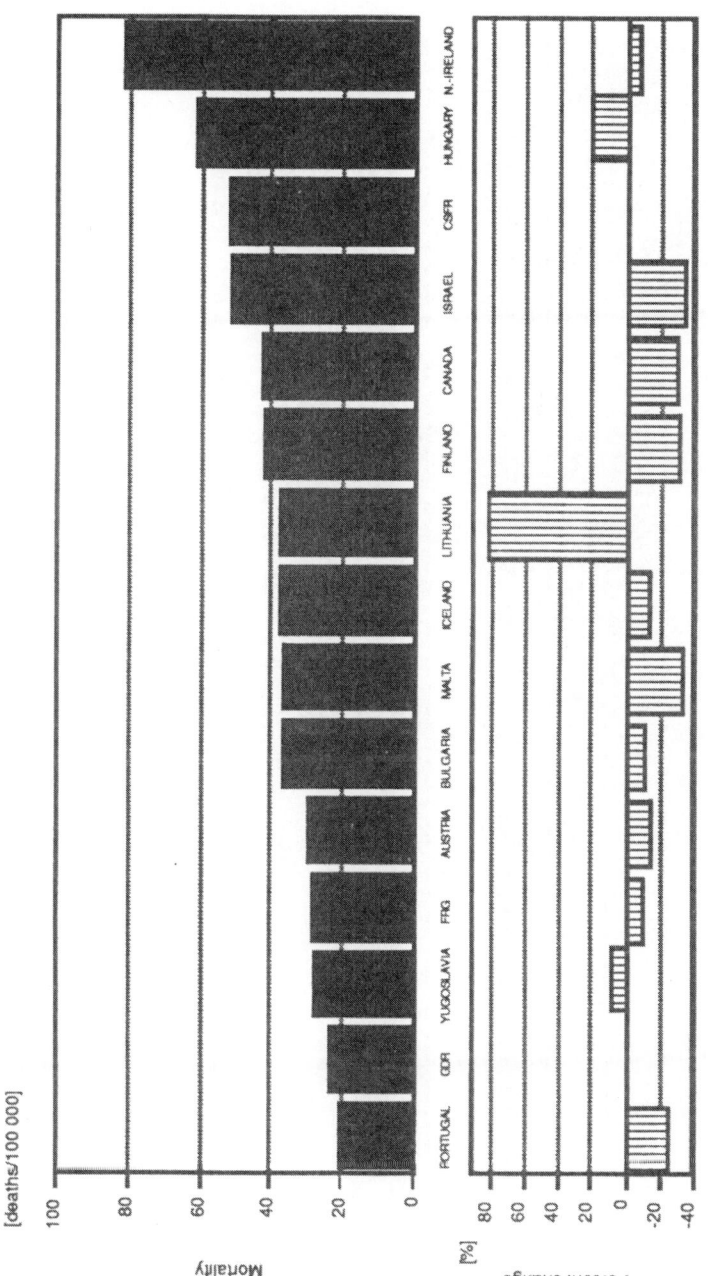

Fig. 6. Age-standardized mortality rates (deaths per 100 000 population) from ischaemic heart disease (ICD 410–414) and percentage change from 1973 to 1982 among women aged 25-64 years.

CSFR, Czech and Slovak Federal Republic; FRG, Federal Republic of Germany before 3 October 1990; GDR, former German Democratic Republic

18

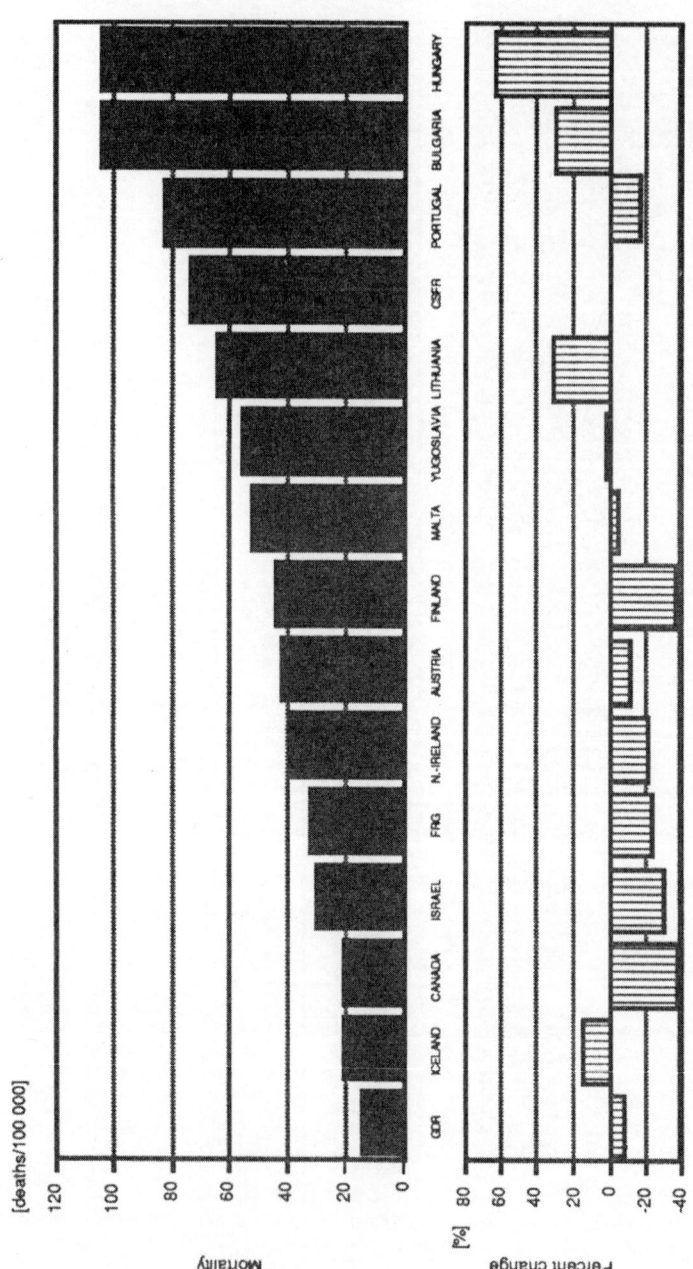

Fig. 7. Age-standardized mortality rates (deaths per 100 000 population) from cerebrovascular disease (ICD 430-438) and percentage change from 1973 to 1982 among men aged 25-64 years.

CSFR, Czech and Slovak Federal Republic; FRG, Federal Republic of Germany before 3 October 1990; GDR, former German Democratic Republic

19

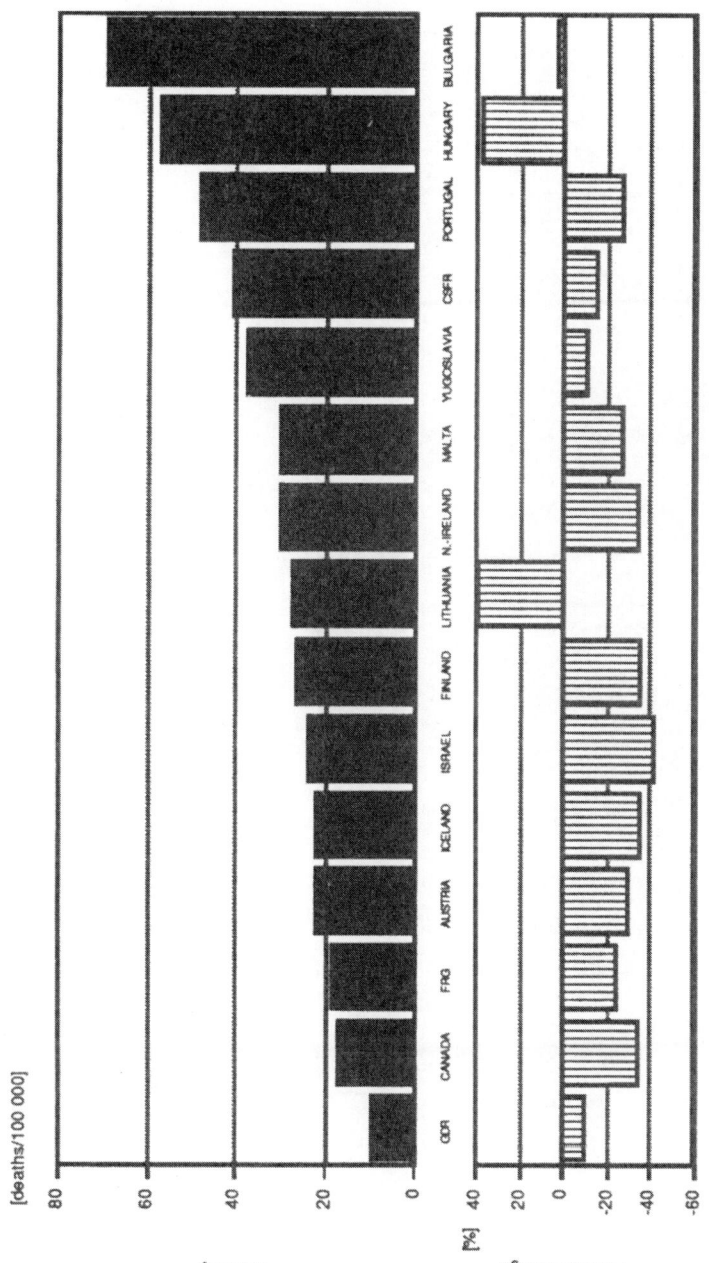

Fig. 8. Age-standardized mortality rates (deaths per 100 000 population) from cerebrovascular disease (ICD 430-438) and percentage change from 1973 to 1982 among women aged 25-64 years.

CSFR, Czech and Slovak Federal Republic; FRG, Federal Republic of Germany before 3 October 1990; GDR, former German Democratic Republic

20

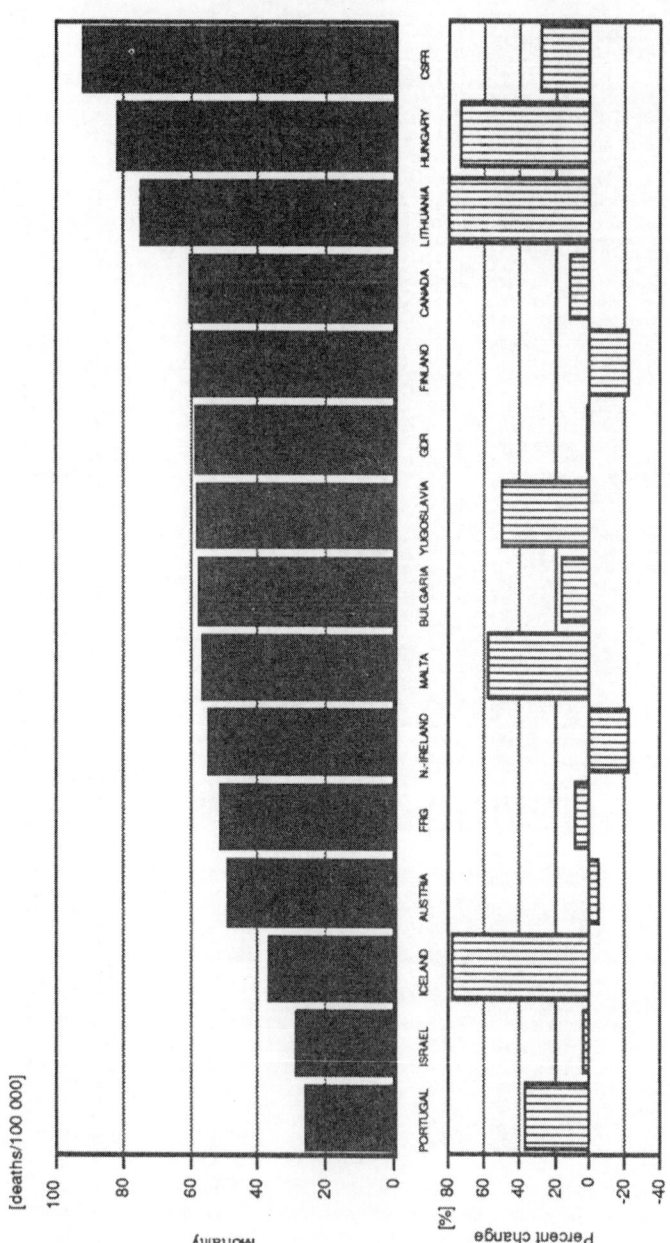

Fig. 9. Age-standardized mortality rates (deaths per 100 000 population) from malignant neoplasms of the trachea, bronchus and lung (ICD 162) and percentage change from 1973 to 1982 among men aged 25-64 years.

CSFR, Czech and Slovak Federal Republic; FRG, Federal Republic of Germany before 3 October 1990; GDR, former German Democratic Republic

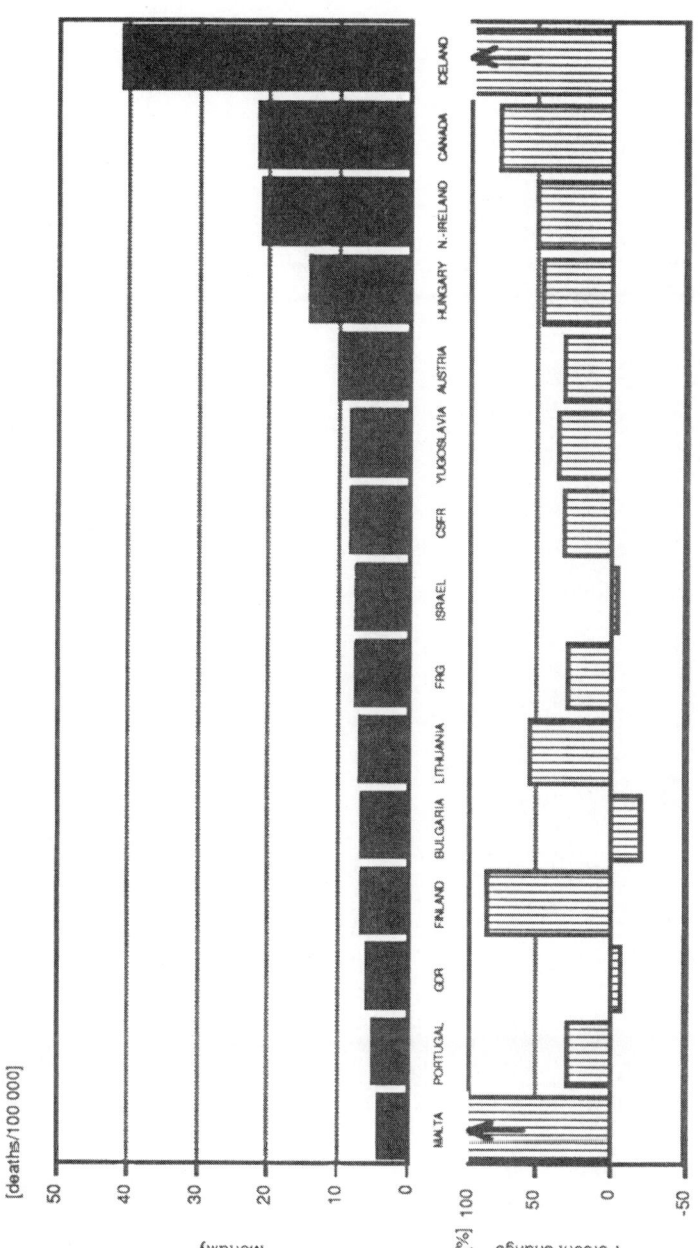

Fig. 10. Age-standardized mortality rates (deaths per 100 000 population) from malignant neoplasms of the trachea, bronchus and lung (ICD 162) and percentage change from 1973 to 1982 among women aged 25-64 years.

CSFR, Czech and Slovak Federal Republic; FRG, Federal Republic of Germany before 3 October 1990; GDR, former German Democratic Republic

22

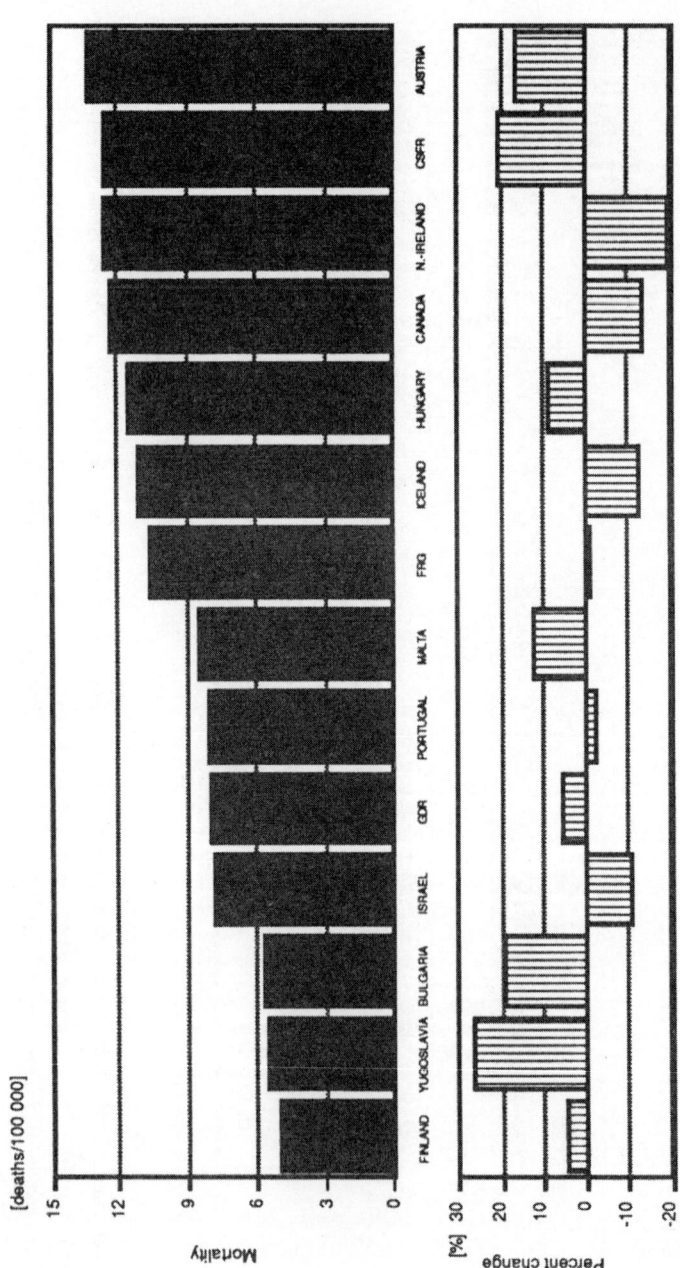

Fig. 11. Age-standardized mortality rates (deaths per 100 000 population) from malignant neoplasms of the small intestine, duodenum and colon (ICD 152–153) and percentage change from 1973 to 1982 among men aged 25-64 years. CSFR, Czech and Slovak Federal Republic; FRG, Federal Republic of Germany before 3 October 1990; GDR, former German Democratic Republic

23

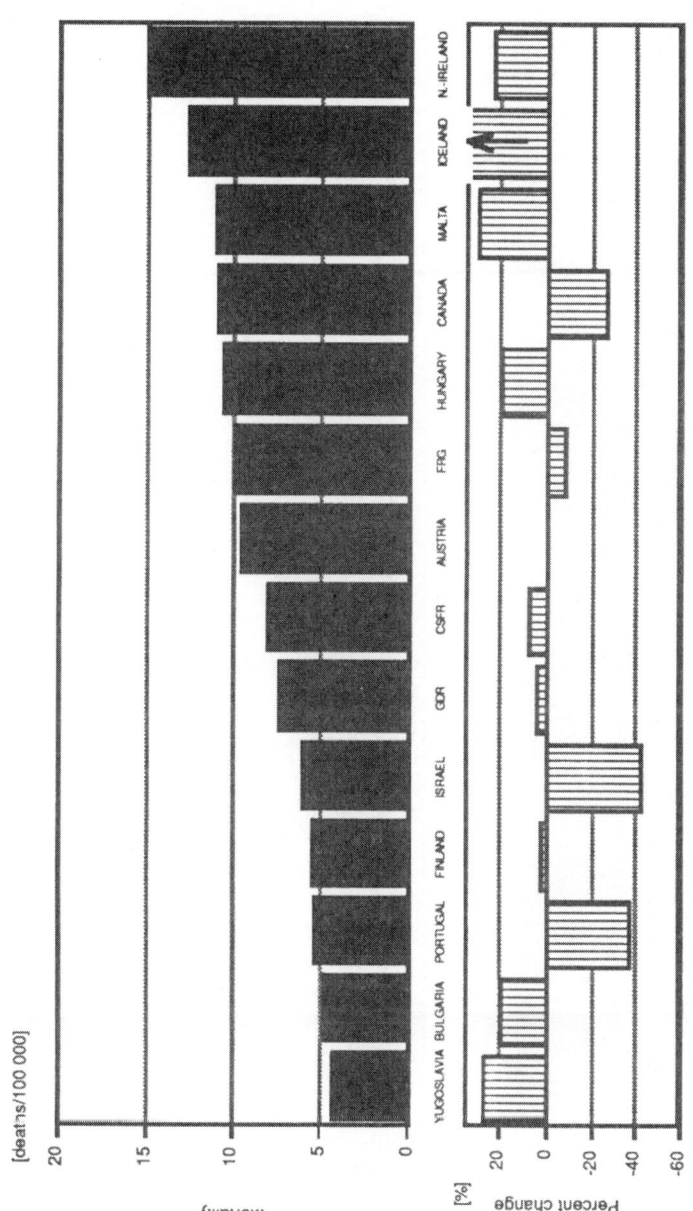

Fig. 12. Age-standardized mortality rates (deaths per 100 000 population) from malignant neoplasms of the the small intestine, duodenum and colon (ICD 152-153) and percentage change from 1973 to 1982 among women aged 25-64 years.

CSFR, Czech and Slovak Federal Republic; FRG, Federal Republic of Germany before 3 October 1990; GDR, former German Democratic Republic

24

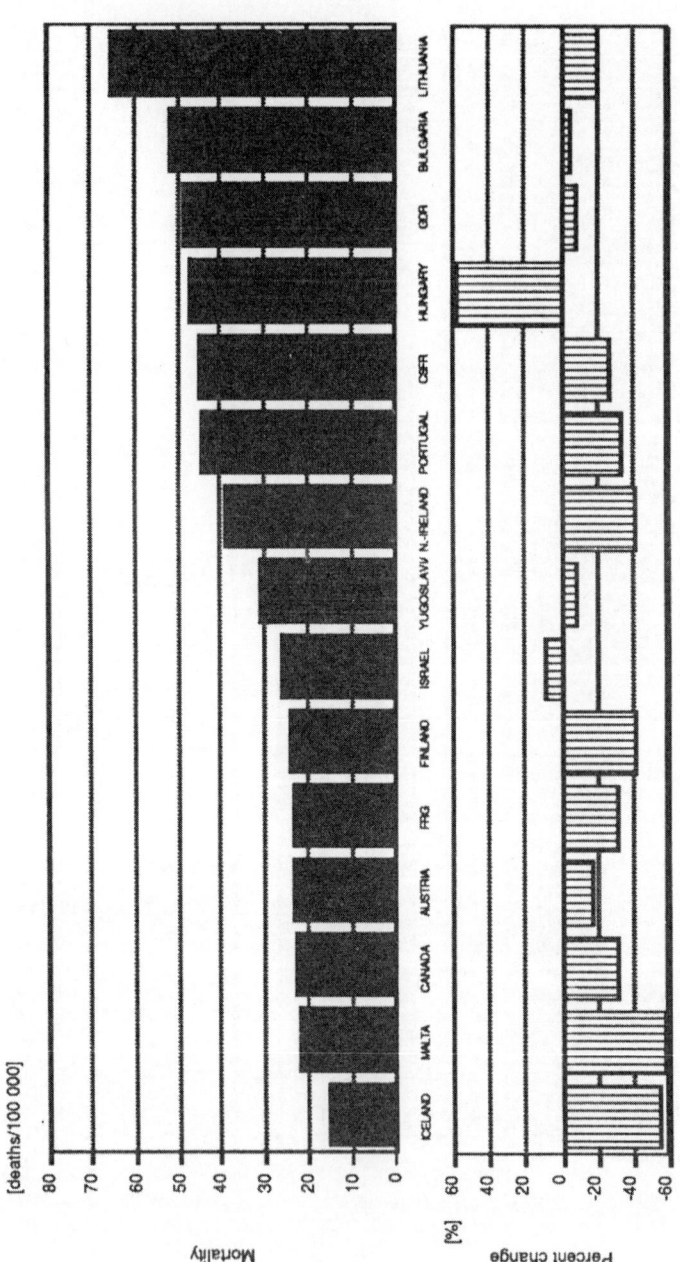

Fig. 13. Age-standardized mortality rates (deaths per 100 000 population) from diseases of the respiratory system (ICD 460-519) and percentage change from 1973 to 1982 among men aged 25-64 years.

CSFR, Czech and Slovak Federal Republic; FRG, Federal Republic of Germany before 3 October 1990; GDR, former German Democratic Republic

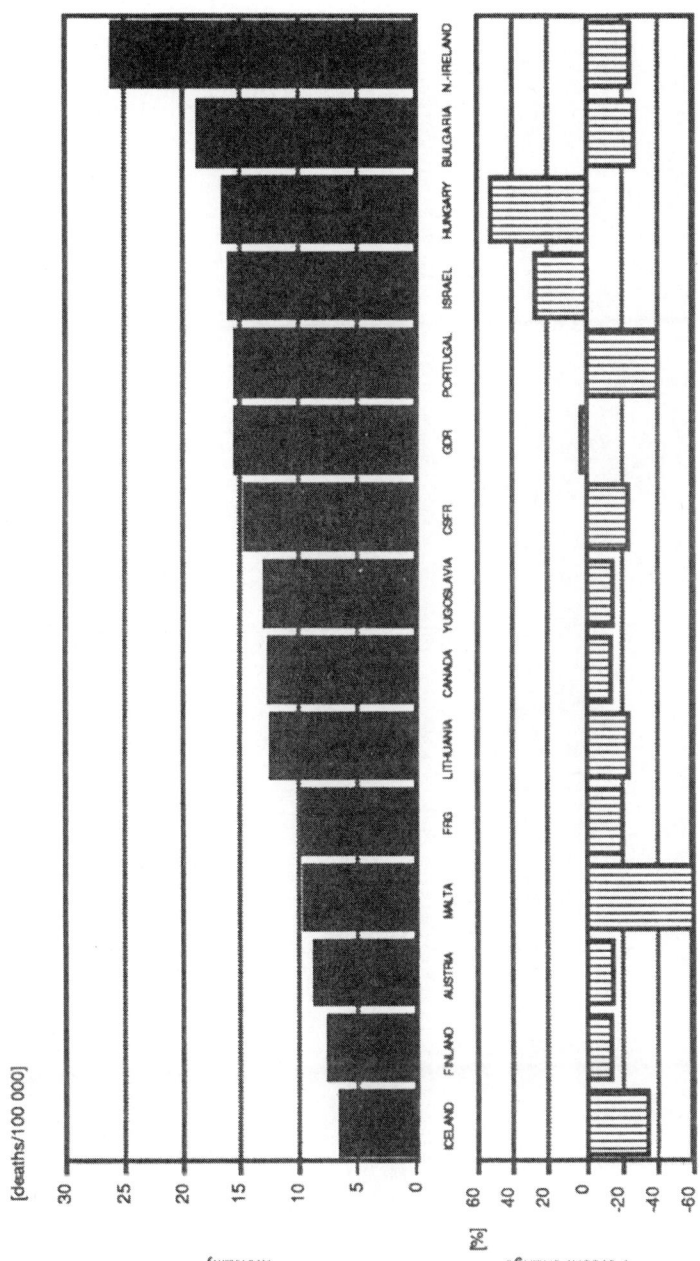

Fig. 14. Age-standardized mortality rates (deaths per 100 000 population) from diseases of the respiratory system (ICD 460-519) and percentage change from 1973 to 1982 among women aged 25-64 years.

CSFR, Czech and Slovak Federal Republic; FRG, Federal Republic of Germany before 3 October 1990 GDR, former German Democratic Republic

25

26

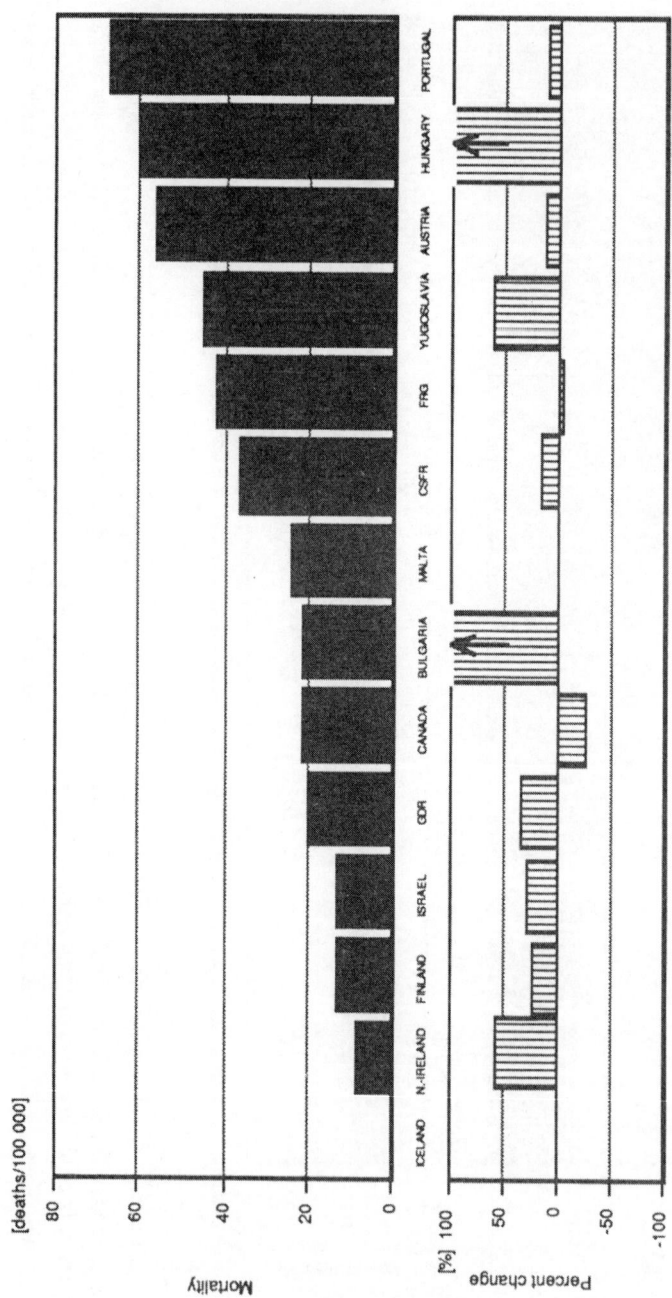

Fig. 15. Age-standardized mortality rates (deaths per 100 000 population) from chronic liver disease and cirrhosis (ICD 571) and percentage change from 1973 to 1982 among men aged 25-64 years.

CSFR, Czech and Slovak Federal Republic; FRG, Federal Republic of Germany before 3 October 1990; GDR, former German Democratic Republic

27

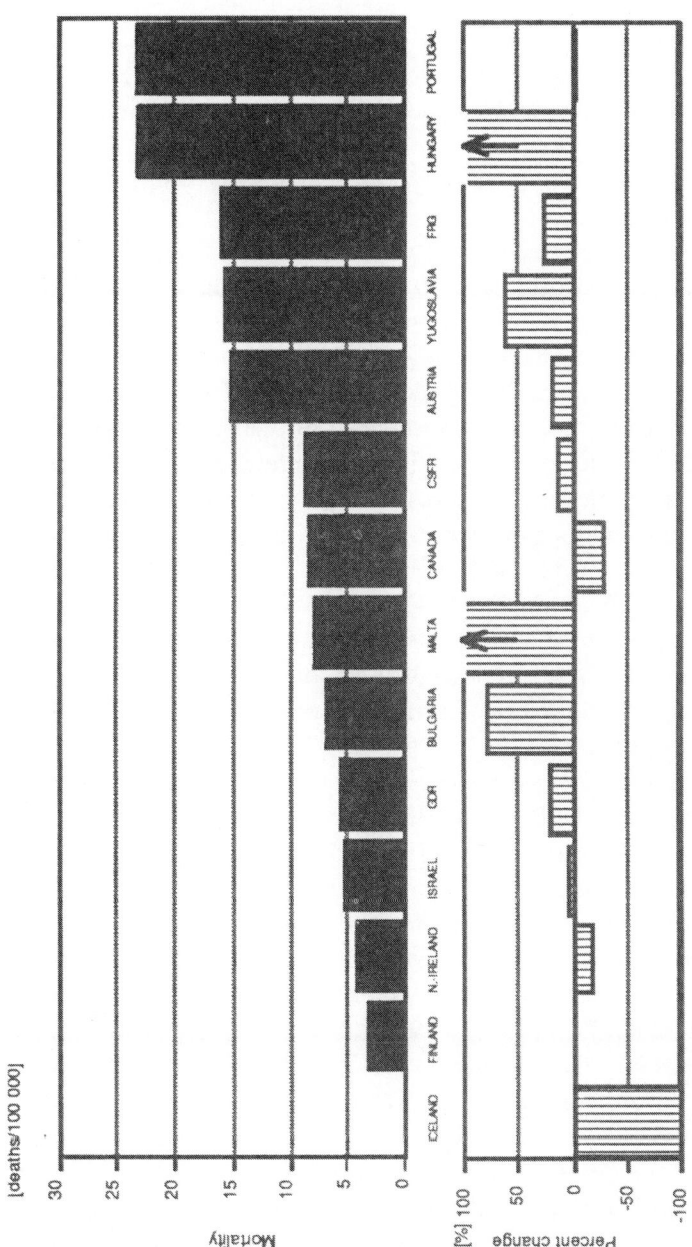

Fig. 16. Age-standardized mortality rates (deaths per 100 000 population) from chronic liver disease and cirrhosis (ICD 571) and percentage change from 1973 to 1982 among women aged 25-64 years.

CSFR, Czech and Slovak Federal Republic; FRG, Federal Republic of Germany before 3 October 1990; GDR, former German Democratic Republic

The risk factor levels constitute an important set of indicators. The data collected by surveys presented here only refer to essential indicators: those defined by the *Guidelines* as mandatory for participation in CINDI. The methods of measurement are described in Annex 7.3. Only CINDI full member countries (Annex 7.1) provide survey data. It is important to note that the surveys only covered random samples in CINDI demonstration areas. Thus, mortality and survey indicators can only be compared by keeping in mind that mortality rates refer to the whole country, whereas survey result indicators may only cover a demonstration area.

Fig. 17 presents data on elevated blood pressure ($\geq$160/95 mmHg) and borderline elevated blood pressure (140-159/90-94 mmHg) among men and women in 13 CINDI countries. In 10 of 13 countries, the age-adjusted prevalence of elevated blood pressure among men was higher than 15%, and in 5 of 13 countries this risk factor was present among more than 20% of the surveyed men (Fig. 17). Canada is the only country that shows a prevalence of elevated blood pressure of under 10%. Four of 13 countries had a prevalence of elevated or borderline elevated blood pressure of more than 50% of the surveyed men.

Eight of 13 countries had a prevalence of elevated blood pressure among women over 15%, versus 10 of the 13 countries among men (Fig. 17). Four countries showed rates higher than 20% for women versus five countries for men. The range of borderline elevated blood pressure prevalence was slightly smaller among women: 11-24% versus 16-30% among men.

The percentage of men with elevated serum cholesterol values ($\geq$250 mg/dl) in the countries ranged between 14% (Canada) and 35% (Finland and Northern Ireland); 6 of 12 countries showed prevalence rates greater then 20% and 4 of 12 countries greater than 30% (Fig. 18). The borderline elevated serum cholesterol (200-249 mg/dl) prevalence was high in all the countries and varied from 32% (Bulgaria) to 49% (GDR).

The prevalence of elevated serum cholesterol was similar among women (Fig. 18) to that among men, varying between 13% (Hungary and Canada) and 35% (Iceland). The percentage of women with borderline elevated cholesterol range between 29% and 47% versus 32-49% for men.

The highest cholesterol values among men and women were observed in Iceland, GDR, Finland, Northern Ireland, FRG and Austria (in decreasing order). The USSR lies in the middle of the distribution. Portugal, Hungary, Canada, Yugoslavia and Bulgaria (in decreasing order) had the lowest cholesterol values (Fig. 18). The rank order for men and women was the same for most countries.

The prevalence of smoking in 12 countries is shown in Fig. 19. Iceland, Canada, Northern Ireland, Finland and GDR were the only countries with prevalence rates lower than 40% for men. Seven other countries had prevalence rates for smoking among men between 40% and 56%. The highest rates were found in eastern Europe (Yugoslavia, USSR and Hungary) and southern Europe (Malta and Portugal).

Women (Fig. 19) had much lower prevalence rates for smoking than men. The rates ranged from 9% in the USSR to 42% in Iceland. Interestingly, three countries with relatively high rates of smoking among men (USSR, Malta and Portugal) had relatively low rates among women, but Yugoslavia had relatively high rates for both genders.

Fig. 20 presents the prevalence of elevated body mass index (BMI) values for men and women, respectively. Elevated BMI values (≥ 30.0 kg/m^2) were more prevalent among women than among men: 11-26% for men versus 13-38% for women, whereas more men than women had elevated or borderline elevated values (>30.0 kg/m^2 or 25.0-29.9 kg/m^2). Malta and Bulgaria had high BMI levels among men and women; Canada had the highest prevalence for men and the USSR for women.

The prevalence of elevated blood pressure, elevated serum cholesterol, smoking and elevated BMI is shown separately for men and women in Fig. 17-20. It is important to determine the prevalence of a combination of risk factors among the population. Fig. 21 presents the proportion of men and women from 11 countries who had no risk factors (see Annex 7.3 for definition) or one or more risk factors. The percentage of men with one or more risk factors ranged between 60% (Canada) and 79% (USSR) and in women between 53% (Portugal) and 71% (Iceland). The rank of the countries was different for men and women.

More than half of the entire population in the CINDI countries is thus burdened with a significantly increased risk of developing noncommunicable diseases.

MEN

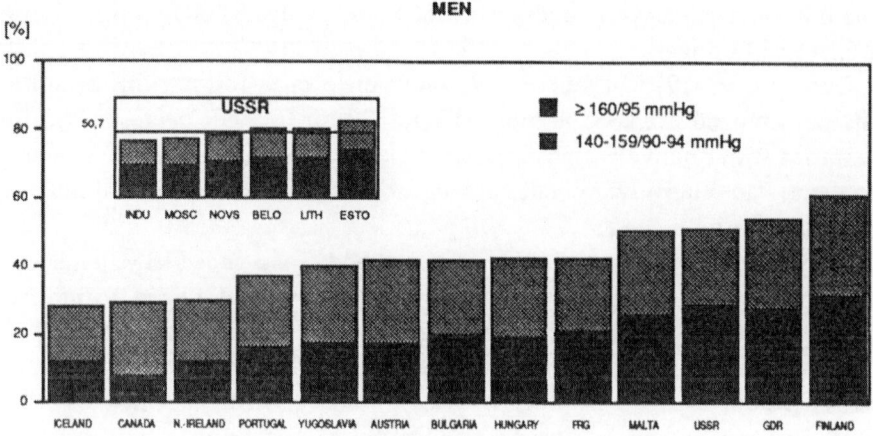

WOMEN

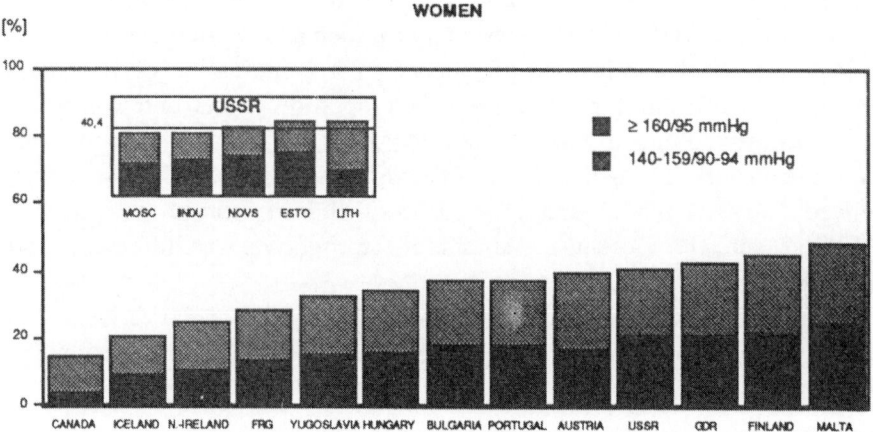

Fig. 17. Age-standardized prevalence (%) of blood pressure ranges among men and women aged 25-64 years.

BELO, Byelorussia (men aged 40-59 years); ESTO, Estonia; FRG, Federal Republic of Germany before 3 October 1990; GDR, former German Democratic Republic; INDU, industrial enterprises; LITH, Lithuania; MOSC, Moscow; NOVS, Novosibirsk

31

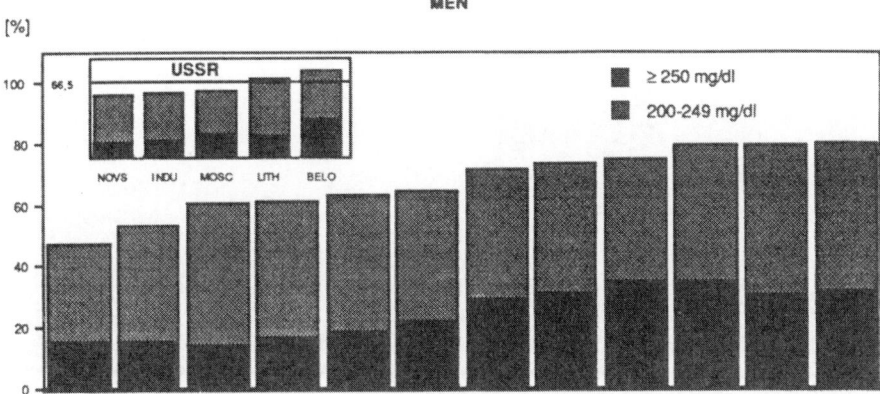

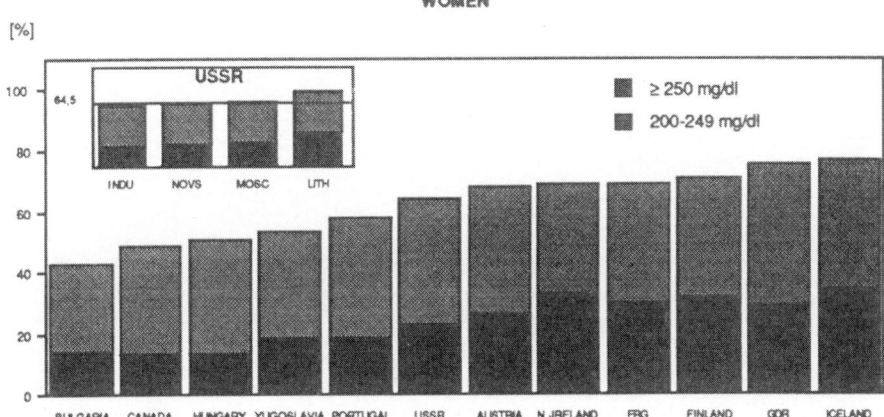

Fig. 18. Age-standardized prevalence (%) of serum cholesterol ranges among men and women aged 25-64 years.

BELO, Byelorussia (men aged 40-59 years); FRG, Federal Republic of Germany before 3 October 1990; GDR, former German Democratic Republic; INDU, industrial enterprises; LITH, Lithuania; MOSC, Moscow; NOVS, Novosibirsk

32

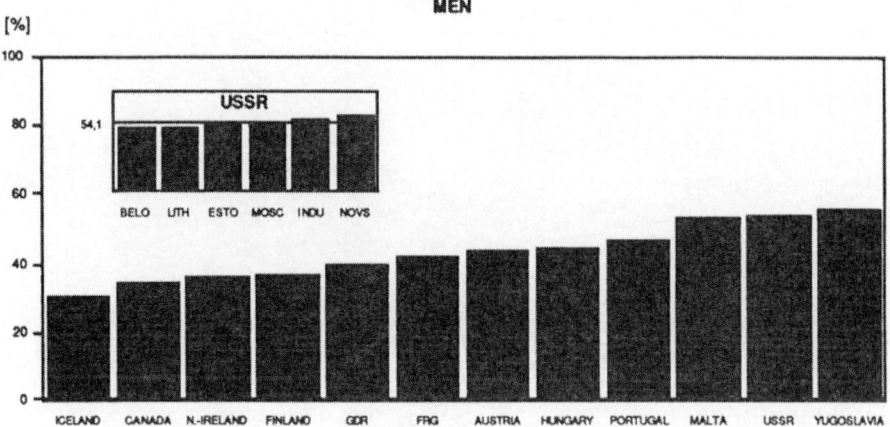

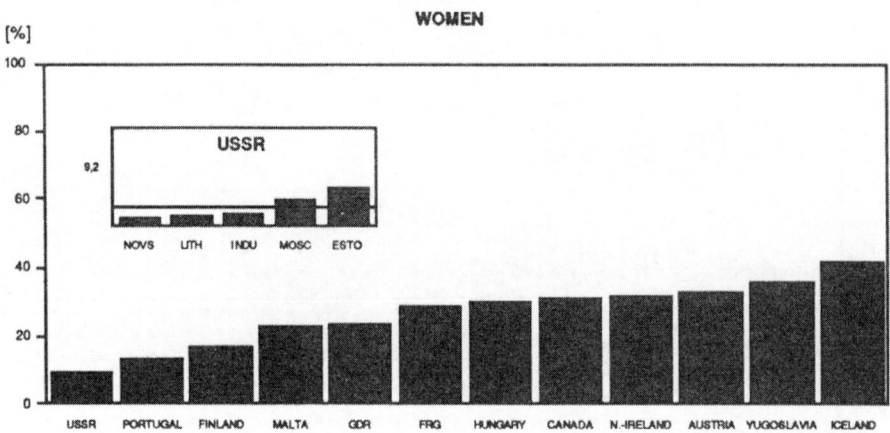

Fig. 19. Age-standardized prevalence (%) of smoking among men and women aged 25-64 years.
BELO, Byelorussia (men aged 40-59 years); ESTO, Estonia; FRG, Federal Republic of Germany before 3 October 1990; GDR, former German Democratic Republic; INDU, industrial enterprises; LITH, Lithuania; MOSC, Moscow; NOVS, Novosibirsk

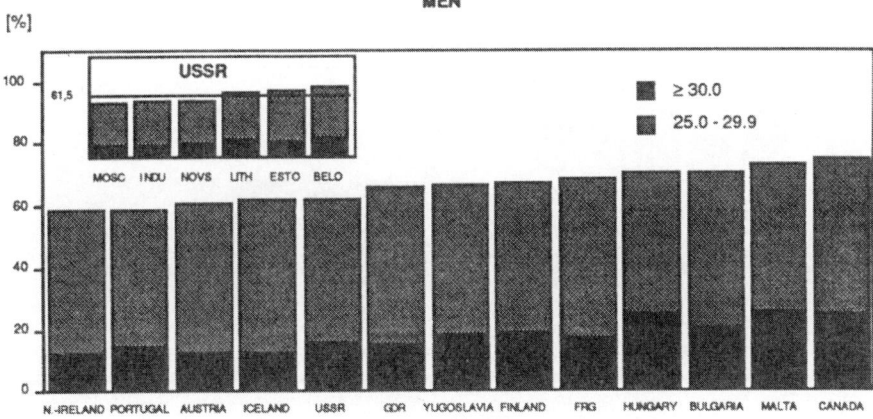

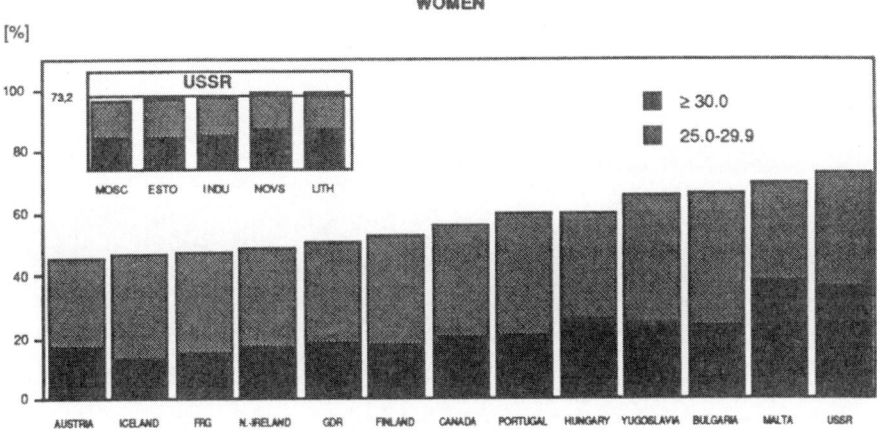

Fig. 20. Age-standardized prevalence (%) of body mass index (kg/m^2) ranges among men and women aged 25-64 years.

BELO, Byelorussia (men aged 40-59 years); ESTO, Estonia; FRG, Federal Republic of Germany before 3 October 1990; GDR, former German Democratic Republic; INDU, industrial enterprises; LITH, Lithuania; MOSC, Moscow; NOVS, Novosibirsk

34

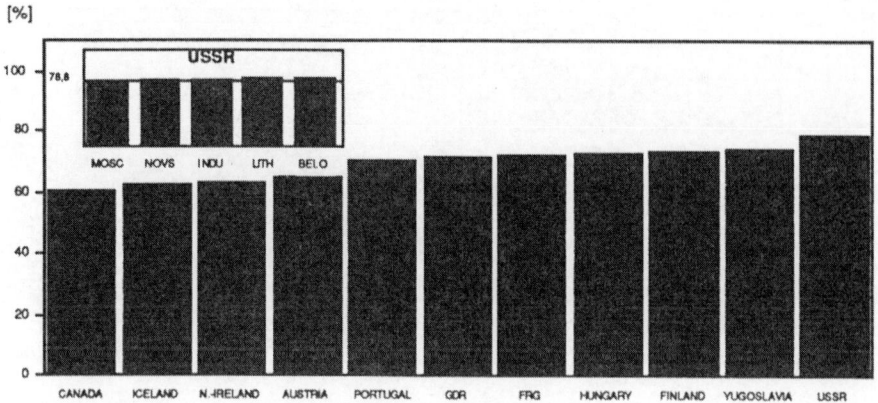

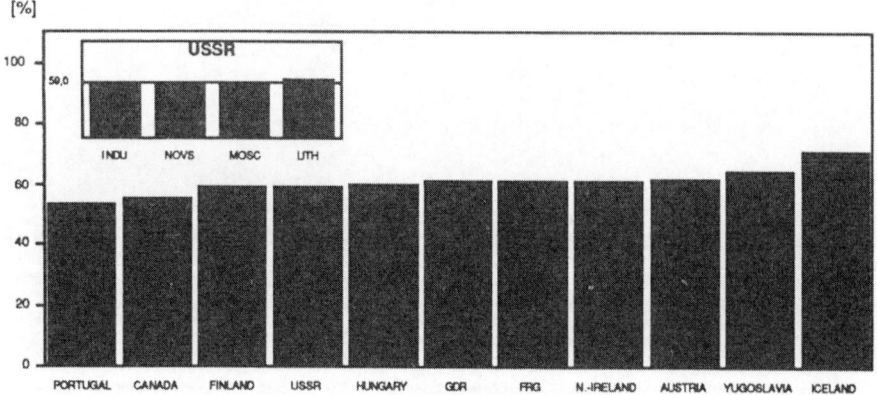

Fig. 21. Age-standardized prevalence (%) of one or more risk factors (serum cholesterol ≥ 250 mg/dl, blood pressure ≥ 160/95 mmHg, BMI ≥ 30 kg/m^2 and smoking) among men and women aged 25-64 years.

BELO, Byelorussia (men aged 40-59 years); FRG, Federal Republic of Germany before 3 October 1990; GDR, former German Democratic Republic; INDU, industrial enterprises; LITH, Lithuania; MOSC, Moscow; NOVS, Novosibirsk

The data presented have several implications. The mortality data from 1982 show many differences between CINDI countries. Trends in mortality rates from noncommunicable diseases differ as well. Some countries in central and eastern Europe had trends towards increasing mortality from cardiovascular diseases (CVD), especially IHD and cerebrovascular disease. At the same time, other European countries and Canada showed a trend towards varying degrees of decline in CVD (mainly IHD and cerebrovascular disease) mortality rates. Countries in eastern Europe should consider adopting a more aggressive and effective approach towards controlling CVD. It is striking that, even in the countries experiencing declining CVD mortality rates, the rates are still high and require attention. Finland and Canada are notable examples.

Some trends are similar in CINDI countries: increasing mortality rates from respiratory cancer and decreasing mortality rates from respiratory diseases not caused by cancer. It is difficult to determine the reasons for these trends, but it can be surmised that the decrease in obstructive respiratory diseases and asthma is related to a decrease in smoking rates in Europe and Canada. The increase in respiratory cancer rates could be related to the high prevalence of smoking in the past, causing death after a time lag.

Another common trend is the increase in mortality rates from chronic liver diseases and cirrhosis of the liver in most CINDI countries. It is difficult to make assumptions about the data, but this phenomenon is probably related to increasing alcohol consumption in these countries.

Common trends might call for a common strategy in the CINDI countries, both in terms of intervention and evaluation, with evaluation results being continually used as feedback for the further development of intervention procedures.

The high level of risk factors found in CINDI surveys is a cause for serious concern. More than 50% of the population - and in some cases up to 70% - has risk factors for noncommunicable diseases. This clearly requires action, not just from the government and public health sector, but also from the population as a whole.

The high prevalence of elevated blood pressure suggests that the measures used to reduce this condition in Europe are clearly insufficient. The situation has improved in Canada, which sets a good example. Smoking rates among men are high everywhere, but lower in Iceland, Northern Ireland and Finland. Elevated serum cholesterol is a universal problem. Obesity is also prevalent in all of the countries.

These data not only justify action, but also imply the need for an informative and continuous system of evaluating indicators of disease and risk factors so that decisions can be made judiciously and appropriate action taken.

5 Additional Baseline Indicators and Plans for Future Development of the Evaluation Framework

In addition to the baseline indicators for the core evaluation referred to in the previous chapter, most countries participating in CINDI use additional indicators that cover younger and older age groups and other causes of death, such as accidents. In most of the countries, risk factor and demographic data also include self-reported presence of diabetes and hypertension, alcohol consumption, physical activity, educational level and marital status. Food consumption data are available for only a few countries.

Indicators of socioeconomic deprivation that are related to the risk of noncommunicable diseases are especially significant for the goals of the CINDI programme and the WHO health for all policy. Differences in mortality from and the risk of cardiovascular disease among different socioeconomic classes within countries have been documented. Reducing inequities in health is an important goal for CINDI programmes, to ensure that the benefits of prevention accrue to all segments of society. CINDI programmes should therefore collect data on indicators of risk for noncommunicable diseases to assess prevention goals properly.

A number of countries participating in CINDI have provided data on the educational level of the survey population. Education is a good indicator of socioeconomic status. Fig. 22 show a more pronounced clustering of risk factors for cardiovascular diseases among people with less education versus people with more education for the countries presented. The risk of cardiovascular disease is inversely related to the level of education. CINDI countries are expected to use this type of analysis more often as the programme develops.

Another way of estimating the CVD risk and the risk of mortality in CINDI populations is to use analytical risk models derived from prospective epidemiological studies. Logistic function models are available that permit the calculation of risk of death from coronary heart diseases and/or death from other causes as a result of the presence of such factors as elevated serum cholesterol, elevated blood pressure, smoking and overweight.

Fig. 23 shows the combined contribution of several CVD risk factors to coronary heart disease mortality within six years for men aged 40-59 years.

38

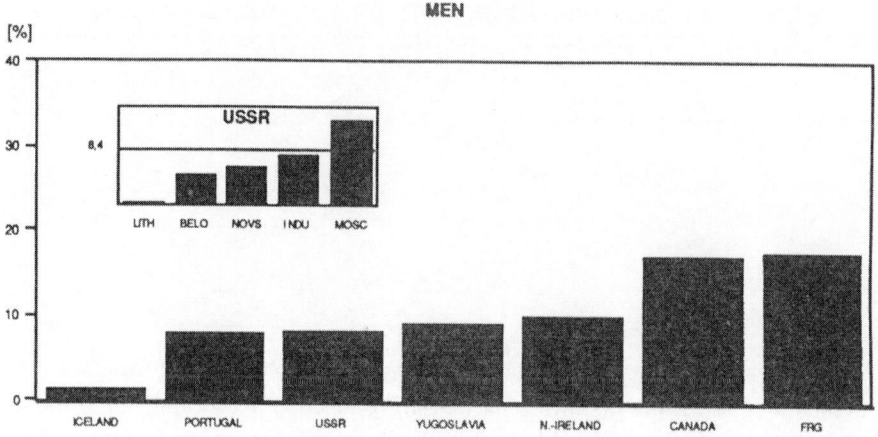

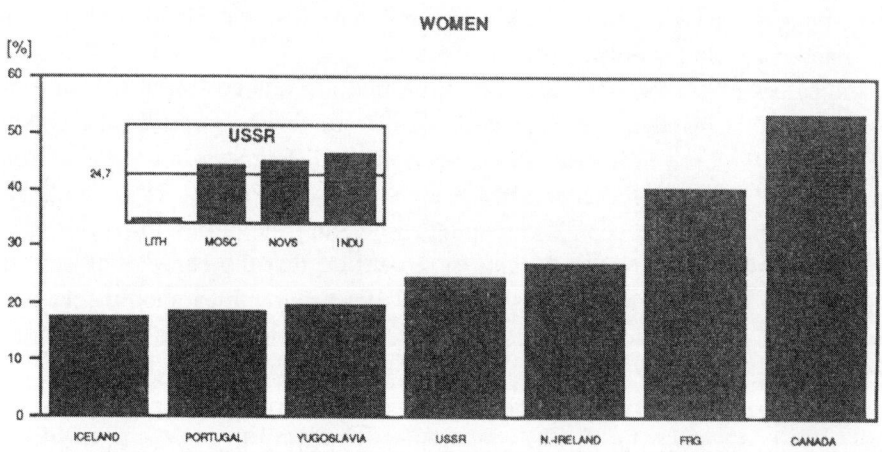

Fig. 22. Differences in age-standardized prevalence of one or more risk factors (serum cholesterol ≥ 200 mg/dl, blood pressure ≥ 140/90 mmHg and smoking) among men and women aged 25-64 years with low and high levels of education expressed as a percentage difference using the percentage of those with higher education as the basis.

BELO, Byelorussia (men aged 40-59 years); FRG, Federal Republic of Germany; INDU, industrial enterprises; LITH, Lithuania; MOSC, Moscow; NOVS, Novosibirsk

The risk is calculated using the risk factor data available from the CINDI country surveys reported in Chapter 4, by means of logistic regression coefficients derived from the prospective components of the WHO project on European risk factors and incidence - a collaborative analysis (ERICA). The estimated risk of coronary heart disease differs markedly; it is relatively high in Finland and Germany and low in Canada and Iceland.

These estimates of CVD risk (Fig. 23) and the continuous rank according to mortality rates for ischaemic heart disease (Fig. 5) should be correlated. This type of comparison requires specific assumptions about the dynamics of change of demographic factors and CVD risk in the population and about how well risk patterns in the demonstration area apply to the country as a whole. The information required for this analysis is not yet readily available. Nevertheless, careful analysis of risk in CINDI programme evaluation and research might be useful in clarifying how well the current levels of CVD risk might predict the future prevalence of diseases and in assessing the value of various intervention strategies.

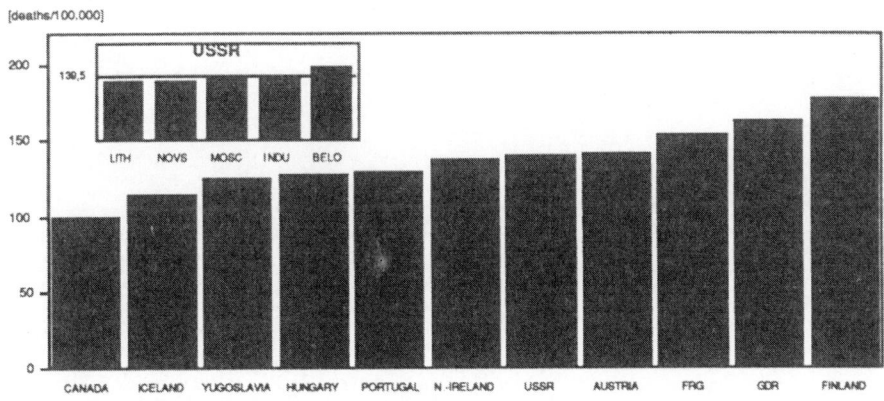

Fig. 23. Multiple risk expressed as estimated coronary heart disease mortality (deaths per 100.000 population) within six years after baseline investigation among men aged 40-59 years. BELO, Byelorussia; FRG, Federal Republic of Germany; GDR, former German Democratic Republic; INDU, industrial enterprises; LITH, Lithuania; MOSC, Moscow; NOVS, Novosibirsk

In addition to the data presented in this report, CINDI programmes may use other important sources of data in establishing baselines for outcome evaluation and in monitoring the prevalence of noncommunicable diseases. The WHO project on monitoring trends and determinants in cardiovascular diseases (MONICA), the WHO ERICA project and the cancer registries available in many CINDI countries are sources of data that complement the core outcome indicators for the CINDI programmes. Ministries of agriculture in CINDI countries and the Food and Agriculture Organization of the United Nations (FAO) are sources of food disappearance data which, subject to certain assumptions, permit the calculation of estimates of nutrient consumption by the population at large.

CINDI programmes are encouraged to use these data sources to implement extended and more complete evaluation models. In the long run, this should enhance the opportunity of comparing programme outcome between countries.

This report focuses on the baseline for long-term epidemiological evaluation of the outcome of the CINDI programme. The *Guidelines* for CINDI programmes also provide for process evaluation, which will be subject of a follow-up baseline report.

6 Implications for Evaluation of CINDI Programmes

The material presented in this report represents the first documentation of the baseline data for the outcome evaluation of the WHO CINDI programme. It is the product of a collaborative effort between participating CINDI countries to coordinate the outcome evaluation of the programmes.

The baseline data show that all CINDI countries face a major challenge in preventing and controlling noncommunicable diseases, which account for the bulk of mortality, morbidity and disability in all the countries.

The inter-country variation in mortality rates and the high levels of risk indicate the potential for prevention that may be achieved by reducing risk in the population at large. Some countries had begun to show favourable trends in ischaemic heart disease and stroke in 1973-1982, before the programme started. In some European countries the mortality rates for these diseases have been increasing, which poses a particular challenge to these countries.

Within countries, the burden of noncommunicable diseases and the level of risk factors vary appreciably according to gender and educational level. This shows that appropriate intervention methods need to be directed towards special groups and different health promotion methods and that disease prevention strategies need to be planned to deal with the cultural and socioeconomic context of risk.

This analysis has concrete implications for the evaluation of CINDI programmes if one of the purposes of outcome evaluation is to assess how well the CINDI programme is meeting its objectives. Countries that have decreasing mortality trends for some noncommunicable diseases, such as ischaemic heart disease, could consider the past rates of reduction as a baseline and strive to accelerate the decline in mortality rates: for example, doubling the annual rate of decline. In contrast, the countries with unfavourable trends may set a target of slowing the rate of increase and eventually reversing the trend.

Inter-country comparisons of prevalence rates may help in setting objectives for intervention programmes to achieve risk reduction. Smoking is a case in point. For example, the prevalence rates for women vary considerably between countries. This suggests a need for different programme approaches and objectives and for expending more resources on assessing the population groups with high prevalence rates, thus maximizing the benefits of programme intervention.

The inter-country differences in secular trends in mortality for the baseline period of 1973-1982 suggest that the dynamics that underlie the observed changes merit further examination. It would be plausible to assume that changes in mortality trends are associated with risk factor trends and with the related socioeconomic determinants. Coordinated evaluation research studies among CINDI member countries and non-members are an important way to determine which of the countries' strategies hold the greatest promise for preventing and controlling major noncommunicable diseases.

The baseline measures of outcome presented in this report are considered to be a minimum core for CINDI programmes.

It is expected that CINDI countries will add to this core, which could support more broadly based evaluation schemes in relation to the years when the programme activities were initiated. Process evaluation, which comprises monitoring programme implementation and how it takes place, is required by the *Guidelines*.

7 Annex

7.1 CINDI Countries and Programme Directors

Full member countries

Austria	Dr H.- P. Bischof and Mag. R. Schiemer
Bulgaria	Professor L. Ivanov
Canada	Dr A. Petrasovits and Dr S. Stachenko
Finland	Professor P. Puska

Federal Republic of Germany

Professor E. Nüssel

German Democratic Republic (until 3 October 1990)

Dr W. Barth

Hungary	Dr A. Szilasi
Iceland	Dr H.V. Fridriksson
Malta	Dr G. Galea
Portugal	Professor F. de Padua
United Kingdom	Professor A.E. Evans and Dr J. Wilde
USSR	Professor R.G. Oganov

44

Yugoslavia   Dr M. Planojevic

Associated countries

Czech and Slovak Federal Republic

                                Dr J. Boukal

Israel   Professor J.R. Viskoper

7.2 CINDI Management Structure

Council of Programme Directors

> Highest policy- and decision-making body for the cooperative CINDI
> programme (see list of programme directors, Annex 7.1).

Programme Management Committee

> Coordinating Centre, Moscow, USSR (Professor G.S. Zhukovsky)
>
> WHO Regional Office for Europe, Copenhagen, Denmark
> (Dr M. Tsechkovski and Dr I. Glasunov)
>
> WHO headquarters, Geneva, Switzerland (Dr E. Chigan)
>
> Data Management Centre, Heidelberg, Federal Republic of Germany
> (Professor E. Nüssel and Mr W. Morgenstern)
>
> CINDI Collaborating Centre, Helsinki, Finland (Professor P. Puska)
>
> Council of Programme Directors (on rotation: for 1991, Dr J. Wilde)

Coordinating Centre:

All-Union Centre for Preventive Medicine, Moscow, USSR

Professor G.S. Zhukovsky

Data Management Centre:

Department of Clinical Social Medicine, University of Ieidelberg, Federal Republic of Germany

Mr W. Morgenstern

7.3 Methods and Data Collection

The data for this publication were processed and analysed by the CINDI Data Management Centre, Heidelberg. The data presented come from CINDI member countries, including the German Democratic Republic, which was a full member before the unification of Germany in 1990.

Mortality data

The basic information for the mortality analysis has been provided by WHO headquarters, Geneva. The CINDI Collaborative Group appreciates this help. The basic information comprises the number of people in a population and the number of deaths according to country, year, gender, and five-year age groups. Additionally, the deaths are classified according to cause in accordance with the International Classification of Diseases (ICD). The data in the WIIO data bank were drawn from the official civil mortality registration system of each country. Data for Lithuania were directly provided by the Lithuanian centre and derive from the official mortality registration system as well.

The data presented are based on the first overall assessment of the baseline in the inter-country evaluation of all CINDI member countries. It could only be carried out from 1988 to 1989 after the deadline of November 1988 for accepting countries as full members. The time period for assessing baseline trends in mortality within countries was defined as the ten-year period from 1973 to 1982, to ensure comparability in the inter-country evaluation during this first stage of analysis. In 1988, most of the CINDI countries' mortality data for 1973-1982 were available at the Data Management Centre (exceptions: German Democratic Republic (1973-1976), Israel (1975-1982), Northern Ireland (1973-1981), Portugal (1973-1981), USSR as a whole (no data) and Yugoslavia (1973-1981).

With the above exceptions, age-standardized mortality rates were calculated for the year 1982 for people aged 25-64 years according to the direct method: a mean of mortality rates for five-year age groups weighted using the European standard population. This reference population is:

Age (years)	Population
25-29	7 000
30-34	7 000
35-39	7 000
40-44	7 000
45-49	7 000
50-54	7 000
55-59	6 000
60-64	5 000

The mortality rates are expressed as deaths per 100 000 population. The percentage change in age-standardized mortality rates between 1973 and 1982 (see exceptions above), which approximately indicates development over time, was calculated as:

$$\frac{R_{1982} - R_{1973}}{R_{1973}} \times 100$$

where R is the age-standardized rate.

Fluctuations in small cause-specific mortality rates (such as those for some malignant neoplasms and chronic liver diseases), especially in countries with small populations (such as Iceland and Malta), should be interpreted cautiously since the variation from year to year is large. For example the mortality rate from malignant neoplasms of trachea, bronchus and lung among women increased in Malta from 0 in 1973 to 4.0 in 1982.

Survey data

Survey data were only provided by CINDI full member countries. Data on anonymous individuals were sent to the Data Management Centre by the CINDI programme directors. The surveys were conducted between 1982 (Finland) and 1987 (Northern Ireland and Portugal) in pilot or demonstration areas (surveys in Iceland and Malta cover the whole country). The USSR reported survey data from pilot or demonstration areas in Byelorussia, Estonia and Lithuania and in the two cities of Moscow and Novosibirsk, as well as survey data on the intervention in industrial enterprises.

Seven of the 18 surveys are identical with the MONICA surveys (Finland, German Democratic Republic, Iceland, Malta, Moscow, Novosibirsk and Yugoslavia). Three surveys cover a greater population than that of their MONICA surveys (Federal Republic of Germany, Lithuania and Northern Ireland). MONICA data from the German Democratic Republic, Iceland, Malta and Lithuania were provided by the MONICA Data Centre, Helsinki. The CINDI Collaborative Group appreciates this help.

The sample sizes for each gender ranged between 604 (Portugal, men) and 4 732 (Finland, women). The surveys were based on simple random sampling procedures (stratified or nonstratified) or cluster sampling in accordance with the *Guidelines*. The participation rates were over 70% in most of the surveys. Altogether, data for 30 843 men and 28 965 women were processed.

The surveys cover the age range 25-64 years for both genders, except for the survey from Byelorussia, which only reported on men 40-59 years old.

The qualified MONICA survey standardization procedures were used as much as possible in the mandatory CINDI evaluation guidelines. The major characteristics of these procedures are (for more detail, see the *Guidelines* and the MONICA manual[1]):

Height, weight: measured without shoes and without heavy garments. Height should be recorded to the nearest centimeter, and weight to the nearest 200 grams.

Smoking: determination is based on a short version of the MONICA standard questionnaire, which may be self-administered.

Serum cholesterol: determination should follow the MONICA standardization procedures, primarily following the external quality control of the WHO Lipid and Reference Centre.

---

[1] WHO MONICA Project (1990) MONICA manual. Unpublished document. Cardiovascular Unit, WHO, Geneva

Blood pressure: measurement after resting in a sitting position and using the
right arm. After 30 seconds, a second measurement. Both
readings should be recorded to the nearest 2 mmHg.

In the Canadian CINDI survey, the standardization procedure of the Lipid
Research Clinics, Atlanta, GA, USA was adopted.

Data for the essential indicators presented in this report are available from
most of the surveys, with the following exceptions (the indicator missing is
given in parentheses): Bulgaria (smoking), Malta (cholesterol) and Estonia
(cholesterol).

The age-standardized prevalence rates were calculated in the same way as
mortality rates: the weighted mean of five-year age-specific prevalence rates.

The cut-off points were defined in accordance with the recommendations of
the European Atherosclerosis Society[1]:

	Normal	Borderline elevated	Elevated
Cholesterol (mg/dl)	< 200	200-249	≥ 250
Blood pressure (mmHg)	< 140/90	140-159/90-94	$\geq 160/95$
BMI (kg/m^2)	< 25.0	25.0-29.9	≥ 30

Smokers were defined as current smokers, not including ex-smokers. The
composite risk was defined as one or more risk factors, which refers to people
who have at least one elevated serum cholesterol, blood pressure or BMI value
or are current smokers.

Multiple risk expressed in estimated coronary heart disease mortality was
calculated as the age-standardized (see above) sum of individual probabilities of
dying from a coronary heart disease event within six years after the baseline
investigation. Individual probabilities were calculated by means of the multiple
logistic risk function published by the ERICA Research Group,[2] which is based
on age, cholesterol, systolic blood pressure, BMI and a dummy variable for
smoking. This risk function was available only for men aged 40-59 years.

---

[1] Study Group of the European Atherosclerosis Society (1987) Strategies for the prevention
of coronary heart disease: a policy statement of the European Atherosclerosis Society. Eur
Heart J 8: 77-78

For each survey, low and high levels of education have been defined according to the data available; categories cannot directly be compared between the individual surveys. They only reflect differences within single survey populations. Differences in prevalence between those with a low level of education and those with a high level of education are expressed as the relative percentage:

$$\frac{PR_{low} - PR_{high}}{PR_{high}} \times 100$$

where PR is the age-standardized prevalence rate.

The data given in the figures for the whole USSR represent the mean of the prevalence observed in each USSR survey population. A small box shows the prevalence in these surveys, with a line representing the mean. For blood pressure, serum cholesterol and BMI, the rates for the elevated and borderline elevated values are combined in calculating this mean.

The exact values of the rates presented in the figures are shown in the tables in Annex 7.4.

7.4 Tables

Table 1. Age-standardized mortality rates per 100 000 population, 1973 and 1982 among men aged 25-64 years

Table 2. Age-standardized mortality rates per 100 000 population, 1973 and 1982 among women aged 25-64 years

Table 3. Age-standardized prevalence (%) among men aged 25-64 years

Table 4. Age-standardized prevalence (%) among women aged 25-64 years

Table 5. Differences in age-standardized prevalence of one or more risk factors (serum cholesterol ≥ 200 mg/dl, blood pressure ≥ 140/90 mmHg and smoking) between individuals with low and high levels of education expressed as a percentage difference using the percentage of those with high education as the basis. Men and women aged 25-64 years

Table 6. Multiple risk expressed as estimated CHD mortality (deaths per 100 000) within a period of 6 years after baseline investigation among men aged 40-59 years

2 ERICA Research Group (1991) Prediction of coronary heart disease in Europe: the 2nd report of the WHO-ERICA project. Eur Heart J 12: 291-297

Table 1. Age-standardized mortality rates per 100 000 population, 1973 and 1982[1] among men aged 25-64 years.
CSFR, Czech and Slovak Federal Republic; FRG, Federal Republic of Germany; GDR, former German Democratic Republic

	Austria	Bulgaria	Canada	CSFR	Finland	FRG	GDR	Hungary	Iceland	Israel	Lithuania	Malta	Northern Ireland	Portugal	Yugoslavia
All causes															
1973	744.7	620.8	703.9	850.2	952.9	724.2	686.9	771.1	608.5	563.6	876.8	756.5	832.1	775.7	734.2
1982	708.1	738.6	581.7	887.6	753.7	634.1	684.7	1044.3	454.2	496.4	1058.7	634.8	693.5	707.8	756.0
Circulatory diseases (ICD 390-459)															
1973	253.0	228.7	305.4	333.8	475.8	251.6	243.3	311.7	237.0	248.3	228.6	345.7	399.6	233.9	220.9
1982	250.4	317.6	228.9	366.2	365.8	231.3	247.8	437.1	191.5	215.3	326.6	327.7	357.5	203.6	255.4
Ischaemic heart diseases (ICD 410-414)															
1973	137.8	101.9	234.9	197.7	342.8	149.9	98.5	155.7	183.5	169.9	129.8	171.3	295.1	80.2	80.7
1982	143.2	129.8	173.5	212.9	276.6	138.8	102.0	239.4	162.7	150.4	207.5	184.0	283.0	75.3	95.5
Cerebrovascular diseases (ICD 430-438)															
1973	47.2	79.9	33.4	74.0	70.2	41.7	16.1	63.7	18.0	42.3	49.0	55.0	50.8	98.8	54.5
1982	41.9	104.0	21.0	74.0	44.3	32.2	14.8	104.2	20.7	30.0	64.2	52.3	39.8	82.5	55.8
All malignant neoplasms (ICD 140-208)[2]															
1973	175.3	148.6	159.5	215.9	182.1	163.3	175.0	180.4	121.0	127.1	177.5	137.6	177.8	141.5	139.4
1982	175.3	162.4	164.3	245.0	155.5	169.0	168.9	236.8	141.7	106.2	215.1	162.9	156.6	145.4	176.7
Malignant neoplasms of trachea, bronchus and lung (ICD 162)															
1973	51.0	49.1	54.5	71.6	75.1	47.3	57.8	46.5	20.5	27.4	41.3	35.2	70.0	19.1	38.0
1982	48.9	57.2	60.7	91.6	59.4	51.4	59.0	81.2	36.7	28.4	74.4	56.3	54.8	26.3	57.6
Malignant neoplasms of intestine, duodenum and colon (ICD 152-153)															
1973	11.4	4.8	14.1	10.3	4.7	10.8	7.5	10.5	12.7	8.8		7.5	15.5	8.2	4.3
1982	13.3	5.7	12.3	12.5	5.0	10.6	8.0	11.5	11.1	7.8		8.4	12.5	8.1	5.5
Respiratory diseases (ICD 460-519)															
1973	28.0	54.7	32.9	61.0	41.1	34.5	52.8	29.5	33.6	23.6	82.1	51.8	65.8	66.8	33.8
1982	23.4	52.0	22.6	44.8	24.4	23.8	48.2	47.3	15.3	25.9	65.4	22.2	39.2	44.5	31.1
Chronic liver diseases and cirrhosis (ICD 571)															
1973	49.8	10.3	28.1	31.3	10.6	42.9	14.6	22.7	0.0	10.2		24.6	5.0	60.2	27.6
1982	56.1	21.3	21.1	36.5	13.1	41.7	20.0	60.4	0.0	13.2		24.0	8.0	66.8	45.2

1 Northern Ireland, Portugal, Yugoslavia (1981), GDR (1976)
2 Lithuania ICD 140-239

Table 2. Age-standardized mortality rates per 100 000 population, 1973 and 1982¹ among women aged 25-64 years. CSFR, Czech and Slovak Federal Republic; FRG, Federal Republic of Germany before 3 October 1990; GDR, former German Democratic Republic

	Austria	Bulgaria	Canada	CSFR	Finland	FRG	GDR	Hungary	Iceland	Israel	Lithuania	Malta	Northern Ireland	Portugal	Yugoslavia
All causes															
1973	367.7	363.0	359.1	401.5	325.3	374.2	385.5	430.7	327.3	394.3	300.3	473.8	454.5	395.3	407.3
1982	320.4	364.7	298.0	378.8	262.1	307.2	372.8	470.0	293.7	306.5	346.1	385.7	382.0	322.9	374.9
Circulatory diseases (ICD 390-459)															
1973	105.7	153.0	107.6	142.7	132.9	93.6	108.5	161.5	92.8	150.0	65.3	177.3	174.1	135.0	132.2
1982	86.4	156.7	77.3	136.7	85.5	76.2	104.1	173.2	68.3	104.1	89.9	130.2	137.6	99.3	137.3
Ischaemic heart diseases (ICD 410-414)															
1973	34.0	40.8	59.1	51.5	60.6	31.2	23.7	50.7	43.4	76.6	20.8	53.8	87.9	27.7	25.2
1982	29.6	36.6	42.5	51.8	42.2	28.3	23.4	61.2	37.9	51.4	37.9	36.8	81.2	21.0	27.5
Cerebrovascular diseases (ICD 430-438)															
1973	31.3	67.5	25.9	48.8	42.2	24.9	11.2	41.4	34.7	41.0	19.9	41.2	45.3	66.6	42.3
1982	22.0	69.4	17.2	41.3	26.9	18.7	10.1	56.9	22.5	24.2	27.6	30.0	30.0	48.1	37.8
All malignant neoplasms (ICD 140-208)²															
1973	142.3	105.1	138.5	140.3	102.7	141.0	135.5	147.8	121.0	134.3	116.5	101.5	152.6	116.8	100.0
1982	131.9	111.3	133.9	140.6	99.3	127.9	134.1	152.1	161.4	111.9	119.6	139.6	154.9	104.7	110.7
Malignant neoplasms of trachea, bronchus and lung (ICD 162)															
1973	7.6	8.5	12.2	6.4	3.6	5.7	6.3	9.7	19.9	8.0	4.6	0.0	14.1	4.0	6.3
1982	10.0	6.8	21.4	8.4	6.6	7.4	5.9	14.1	40.6	7.7	7.1	4.0	21.2	5.2	8.6
Malignant neoplasms of intestine, duodenum and colon (ICD 152-153)															
1973	9.7	4.0	14.8	7.4	5.4	10.7	7.2	8.9	2.7	10.7		8.5	12.0	8.6	3.4
1982	9.6	4.8	10.9	8.0	5.5	9.9	7.4	10.6	12.6	6.1		11.1	14.9	5.4	4.3
Respiratory diseases (ICD 460-519)															
1973	10.3	25.5	14.5	18.7	8.7	12.3	14.9	10.7	10.1	12.4	16.2	23.8	34.8	25.3	15.1
1982	8.8	18.6	12.5	14.5	7.6	9.8	15.4	16.4	6.6	15.9	12.4	9.5	26.0	15.5	12.8
Chronic liver diseases and cirrhosis (ICD 571)															
1973	12.5	3.7	11.4	7.4	3.3	12.3	4.5	8.1	2.4	4.9		3.5	4.8	24.0	9.5
1982	15.0	6.6	8.3	8.4	3.2	15.7	5.5	22.9	0.0	5.1		7.7	4.0	23.2	15.5

¹ Northern Ireland, Portugal, Yugoslavia (1981), GDR (1976)
² Lithuania ICD 140-239

Table 3. Age-standardized prevalence (%) among men aged 25-64 years.

FRG, Federal Republic of Germany before 3 October 1990; GDR, former German Democratic Republic

	Austria	Bulgaria	Canada	Finland	FRG	GDR	Hungary	Iceland	Malta	Northern Ireland	Portugal	USSR						Yugo-slavia
												Byelo-russia[2]	Estonia	Industrial enterprises	Lithuania	Moscow	Novo-sibirsk	
Serum cholesterol																		
n	683	1695	636	4614	2799	1084	919	827	947	1829	598	3201		1935	1198	531	1374	789
< 200 mg/dl	28.2	52.9	39.8	20.8	26.4	20.4	38.4	19.9	49.4	25.2	35.4	20.0		39.7	28.0	37.7	42.0	47.0
200-249 mg/dl	42.9	31.7	46.3	44.0	42.2	49.1	44.9	47.7	24.8	39.7	42.4	44.4		43.2	50.6	39.7	43.6	38.1
≥ 250 mg/dl	29.0	15.4	13.9	35.2	31.4	30.5	16.6	32.4	25.8	35.1	22.2	35.6		17.1	21.4	22.5	14.4	15.0
Blood pressure																		
n	686	1716	633	4605	2782	1110	1203	828	933	1872	601	4154	794	3834	1252	799	1552	801
< 140/90 mmHg	58.5	58.3	71.1	38.4	57.4	45.8	57.6	72.0	28.1	70.5	63.1	48.1	39.7	56.2	46.9	54.4	51.3	61.0
140-159/90-94 mmHg	24.6	22.2	20.7	29.5	22.0	27.2	23.3	15.8	46.9	17.5	21.1	21.3	23.1	20.2	21.5	22.8	21.6	22.0
≥ 160/95 mmHg	16.9	19.6	8.2	32.1	20.6	27.0	19.1	12.2	25.0	12.0	15.9	30.7	37.2	23.6	31.7	22.8	27.1	17.0
Body mass index																		
n	686	1716	636	4609	2800	1106	1204	827		1161	591	4143	794	3777	1245	768	1552	801
< 25.0 kg/m²	40.0	29.8	23.7	33.8	32.1	35.1	30.3	38.6		41.4	41.4	29.4	34.5	43.7	35.7	45.5	42.6	34.2
25.0-29.9 kg/m²	48.4	50.5	50.7	48.0	51.6	50.2	46.0	50.1		47.2	45.0	49.9	49.4	44.2	45.6	43.2	44.6	48.2
≥ 30.0 kg/m²	11.5	19.7	25.6	18.2	16.3	14.6	23.8	11.4		11.4	13.6	20.7	16.1	12.1	18.7	11.3	12.9	17.6
Smoking																		
n	907		731	4441	2799	1114	1204	827	1008	1870	604	4151	794	3821	1252	799	1552	945
no	56.5		65.5	63.0	57.5	60.3	55.8	69.4	46.1	63.8	53.0	49.8	47.8	41.1	49.5	47.3	39.8	44.2
yes	43.4		34.5	37.0	42.5	39.7	44.2	30.6	53.9	36.2	47.0	50.2	52.2	58.9	50.5	52.7	60.2	55.8
Risk factors[1]																		
n	606		633	4426	2752	1072	918	825		1136	587	3193		1877	1192	531	1374	789
none	35.4		39.8	26.4	28.0	28.5	27.3	37.5		36.3	29.2	18.5		20.7	19.4	26.4	21.2	25.7
one or more	64.6		60.2	73.6	72.0	71.5	72.7	62.5		63.7	70.8	81.5		79.3	80.6	73.6	78.8	74.3

1 smoking, serum cholesterol ≥ 250 mg/dl, blood pressure ≥ 160/95 mmHg, BMI ≥ 30 kg/m²

2 men aged 40-59 years

Table 4. Age-standardized prevalence (%) among women aged 25-64 years.

FRG, Federal Republic of Germany before 3 October 1990; GDR, former German Democratic Republic

	Austria	Bulgaria	Canada	Finland	FRG	GDR	Hungary	Iceland	Malta	Northern Ireland	Portugal	USSR Estonia	USSR Industrial enterprises	USSR Lithuania	USSR Moscow	USSR Novosibirsk	Yugoslavia
Serum cholesterol																	
n	727	3161	687	4726	2885	1176	896	916	930	1862	709		2173	1254	544	1423	777
< 200 mg/dl	31.7	56.9	51.2	28.6	30.0	24.5	48.7	22.5	52.1	31.0	42.0		40.5	27.7	35.8	37.9	46.8
200-249 mg/dl	42.0	28.9	35.6	39.2	39.1	46.5	38.5	43.0	23.8	36.2	39.1		40.3	41.4	41.1	40.7	34.6
≥ 250 mg/dl	26.3	14.1	13.2	32.2	30.1	29.0	12.8	34.5	24.1	32.8	18.9		19.1	30.8	23.1	21.4	18.6
Blood pressure																	
n	727	3200	683	4724	2873	1227	1198	917		1925	711	834	3843	1329	800	1589	781
< 140/90 mmHg	60.9	63.8	85.9	55.6	72.1	58.0	66.0	80.3		76.4	63.4	56.7	62.9	56.0	63.0	59.4	68.1
140-159/90-94 mmHg	22.4	19.1	10.6	22.9	15.0	21.7	18.5	11.4		13.6	19.6	17.5	16.9	28.6	18.8	16.9	17.6
≥ 160/95 mmHg	16.7	17.1	3.6	21.5	12.9	20.3	15.5	8.3		10.0	17.0	25.8	20.2	15.4	18.2	23.7	14.3
Body mass index																	
n	727	3199	687	4729	2889	1217	1199	918	920	1200	696	834	3792	1319	766	1589	781
< 25.0 kg/m²	54.5	33.8	44.1	47.6	53.0	49.2	40.0	53.7	30.2	51.6	40.3	29.2	27.5	21.8	32.6	23.0	34.0
25.0-29.9 kg/m²	29.1	42.1	35.7	34.6	31.4	32.6	34.0	33.4	31.4	31.7	38.7	38.6	37.5	36.9	35.7	36.7	40.8
≥ 30.0 kg/m²	16.5	24.0	20.1	17.8	15.6	18.2	26.0	12.9	38.4	16.8	20.9	32.3	35.0	41.3	31.7	40.2	25.1
Smoking																	
n	865		792	4608	2879	1229	1209	918	1032	1931	712	834	3839	1330	800	1589	896
no	67.8		69.1	83.2	71.3	76.6	69.9	58.0	77.8	68.3	86.7	80.2	94.0	95.9	88.0	96.1	64.0
yes	32.2		30.9	16.8	28.7	23.4	30.1	42.0	22.2	31.7	13.3	19.8	6.0	4.1	12.0	3.9	36.0
Risk factors [1]																	
n	601		683	4591	2828	1163	896	915		1152	694		2126	1245	544	1423	777
none	38.3		44.5	41.1	38.6	38.7	40.5	28.7		38.6	46.7		43.7	35.5	42.3	42.4	35.2
one or more	61.7		55.5	58.9	61.4	61.3	59.5	71.3		61.4	53.3		56.3	64.5	57.7	57.6	64.8

[1] smoking, serum cholesterol ≥ 250 mg/dl, blood pressure ≥ 160/95 mmHg, BMI ≥ 30 kg/m²

54

Table 5. Differences in age-standardized prevalence of one or more risk factors (serum cholesterol ≥ 200 mg/dl, blood pressure ≥ 140/90 mmHg and smoking) between individuals with low and high levels of education expressed as a percentage difference using the percentage of those with high education as the basis. Men and women aged 25-64 years.

FRG, Federal Republic of Germany before 3 October 1990

| | Canada | FRG | Iceland | Northern Ireland | Portugal | Byelorussia¹ | USSR | | | | Yugoslavia |
							Industrial enterprises	Lithuania	Moscow	Novosibirsk	
Men	17.6	17.7	1.7	10.4	8.3	6.1	10.2	0.6	17.0	7.9	9.4
Women	53.7	40.6	17.6	26.9	18.6		34.8	2.1	30.1	31.6	19.5

¹ men aged 40-59 years

Table 6. Multiple risk expressed as estimated CHD mortality (deaths/100 000) within a period of 6 years after baseline investigation among men aged 40-59 years.

FRG, Federal Republic of Germany before 3 October 1990; GDR, former German Democratic Republic

| Austria | Canada | Finland | FRG | GDR | Hungary | Iceland | Northern Ireland | Portugal | Byelorussia | Industrial enterprises | USSR | | | Yugoslavia |
											Lithuania	Moscow	Novosibirsk	
141.5	101.1	176.7	152.8	161.6	128.2	115.7	136.6	130.1	162.6	141.5	123.5	135.9	128.9	126.0